D1446602

PSYCHIATRIC DISORDER and the URBAN ENVIRONMENT

Report of the Cornell Social Science Center

SOCIAL PROBLEMS SERIES
Sheldon R. Roen, Editor

Program Evaluation in the Health Fields
Edited by Herbert C. Schulberg, Ph.D., Alan Sheldon, M.D., and
Frank Baker, Ph.D.

**Psychiatric Disorder and the Urban Environment: Report of the Cornell
Social Science Seminar**
Edited by Berton H. Kaplan, Ph.D. in collaboration with Alexander
H. Leighton, M.D., Jane Murphy, Ph.D., and Nicholas Freydberg,
Ph.D.

**Research, Planning, and Action for the Elderly: The Power and
Potential of Social Science**
Edited by Donald Kent, Ph.D., Robert Kastenbaum, Ph.D., and
Silvia Sherwood, Ph.D.

**Crises of Family Disorganization: Programs to Soften their Impact on
Children**
Edited by Eleanor Pavenstedt, M.D. and Viola W. Bernard, M.D.

Retirement
Frances M. Carp, Ph.D.

Identifying Suicide Potential
Edited by Dorothy B. Anderson and Lenora J. McClean

Two, Four, Six, Eight, When You Gonna Integrate?
Frank A. Petroni and Ernest A. Hirsch with C. Lillian Petroni

PSYCHIATRIC DISORDER and the URBAN ENVIRONMENT

Report of the Cornell Social Science Center

Berton H. Kaplan, Ph.D., Editor
University of North Carolina, Chapel Hill

in collaboration with
Alexander H. Leighton, M.D.
Harvard School of Public Health, Boston
Jane M. Murphy, Ph.D.
Harvard School of Public Health, Boston
and
Nicholas Freydberg, Ph.D.
Payne-Whitney Clinic, New York Hospital, New York

Behavioral Publications   New York

79977

Library of Congress Catalog Card Number 77-140050
Standard Book Number 87705-020-1
Copyright © 1971 by Behavioral Publications

BEHAVIORAL PUBLICATIONS, 2852 Broadway—Morningside Heights,
New York, New York 10025

Printed in the United States of America

To Ellen, Daniel, and Ron and to the ancient
hope for peace and justice in human affairs.

B.H.K.

The Cornell Social Science Seminar Series on Psychiatric Disorder and the Urban Environment was directed by Alexander H. Leighton, M.D.

This work was conducted as a part of the Cornell Program in Social Psychiatry, Department of Psychiatry of New York Hospital, Cornell University Medical College, and Department of Sociology of the College of Arts and Sciences, Cornell University, 1965-66. Funds were provided by Public Health Service Grant 08180, Alexander H. Leighton, M.D., principal investigator. The editor, Berton H. Kaplan, Ph.D., was a Social Science Research Council Fellow during the period of this work. The grantors are not, of course, the authors, owners, publishers or proprietors of this report and are not to be understood as approving, by virtue of their grants, any of the statements made or views expressed herein.

Contents

Contributors and
Seminar Participants

Lloyd Brightman, Ph.D.

Isidor Chein, Ph.D.

Catherine Fales, M.D.

Harold Feldman, Ph.D.

John R. P. French, Jr., Ph.D.

Nicholas Freydberg, Ph.D.

Herbert Gans, Ph.D.

John Gulick, Ph.D.

Paul V. Gumpl, Ph.D.

John S. Harding, Ph.D.

Lawrence E. Hinkle, Jr., M.D.

Laurel Hodgden, Ph.D.

Raymond Illsley, Ph.D.

Mirra Komarovsky, Ph.D.

Thomas Langner, Ph.D.

Alexander H. Leighton, M.D.

Dorothea C. Leighton, M.D.

Stanley T. Michael, M.D.

Jane M. Murphy, Ph.D.

William F. Whyte, Ph.D.

Preface

Alexander H. Leighton, M.D., at that time Director of the Cornell Program in Social Psychiatry (now Chairman of the Department of Behavioral Science at the Harvard School of Public Health), originated and guided the Cornell Social Science Seminar on Psychiatric Disorder and the Urban Environment. The basic orienting question for the seminar study group was as follows: What are the strategy alternatives for studying the urban environment's influence on mental health and mental illness? This basic question stemmed from the work of Leighton as director of the Stirling County Series and, after the death of Thomas A. C. Rennie, as the director of the Midtown Study. In fact, in Chapter 2, Leighton provides a natural history of his long professional interest in the impact of culture on personality.

With the experience gained in the two landmark psychiatric epidemiologic studies, the Stirling County Study and the Midtown Study, the time had come to pause and take a look at "what next?" The "what next" question then gave rise to a special seminar series on psychiatric disorder and the urban environment. Some of the proceedings of the seminar have been pulled together in this summarizing document.

In the development of this manuscript, I am very indebted to the excellent advice and unfailing support of Alexander H. Leighton, Alice Nangeroni, Jane M. Murphy, Nicholas Freydberg, William Foote Whyte, Robin Williams, and Robert N. Wilson. Any deficiencies in this document are, of course, my own responsibility.

I must give very special thanks and credit to Nicholas Freydberg. He wrote the seminar summaries and edited many of the original transcripts from the seminar.

It is very important to point out our rationale for developing this special kind of book: a. to preserve the exchange of ideas that appeared most relevant to the future development of the field of social psychiatry; b. to stimulate the clarification of ideas on social processes and mental illness; c. to preserve some worthwhile ideas and information that otherwise would be fugitive; and d. to preserve selected commentaries that illustrate how experienced investigators have asked various questions on studying the impact of social processes on mental health.

One final comment. The coverage of ideas in this book is not intended to be comprehensive although important contributions for future testing and improvement are preserved and presented.

Berton H. Kaplan, Ph.D.
July, 1970

1

Introduction

BERTON H. KAPLAN, Ph.D.

I intend this chapter to be of some help in considering how to read the book. Its format is based on the following considerations: (a) that the current statement of Alexander Leighton's theory of integration-disintegration should be presented; (b) that a current statement of the empirical status of Leighton's theory should follow; (c) that the seminar critiques and assessments should be included; and (d) that the strategy alternatives for implementing Leighton's frame of reference in urban settings should be presented.

These considerations were implemented in the following way. In Chapter 2, Alexander H. Leighton provides a background statement on how his interest in the relationships between culture and mental health developed in his life-long interest in integration and disintegration as crucial factors in mental illness.

In Chapter 3, Jane M. Murphy states the seminar objectives in precise terms. Her paper illustrates the key questions posed for the seminar. How do we develop conceptual and methodological rigor about the relationship between social processes and mental health? In Chapter 4, the theory of integration-disintegration is outlined and discussed by its originator, Alexander H. Leighton. This chapter is an up-to-date statement by him of his long work on the problems of integration-disintegration, which culminated in the classic, *My Name is Legion* [1].

[1] Leighton, Alexander H. *My name is legion.* New York: Basic Books, 1959.

Next, in Chapter 5, the empirical status of the ten basic hypotheses of Leighton's integration-disintegration theory is reviewed by Dorothea C. Leighton.

In Chapter 6, utilizing the discussions that took place in the Cornell Social Science Seminar, we have a critical review of the integration-disintegration theory. This review consists of the following: the various dimensions of integration-disintegration that were explored in the discussions; four different summaries of the concept of integration-disintegration; and John French's critical commentary on the entire integration-disintegration frame of reference. The reader finds here a searching examination of the problem of clarifying social process influences on mental health.

The remainder of this book, based on the seminar discussions, provides a series of alternate research questions and conceptual schemes for studying social processes and mental illness, particularly in urban settings.

In Chapter 7, Isidor Chein presents his observations on how to use socio-demographic indices to study mental health in urban settings. Several questions dominated the seminar discussions on urban indicators. How can socio-demographic indices be used in an urban setting to study integration and disintegration? What specific social processes should be studied, e.g., within the family, work settings? Why do some people break down in integrated settings? What is there about disintegrated settings that interferes with need-meeting activities?

The next two chapters, 8 and 9, consist of the presentations on the family made to the seminar by Harold Feldman and Mirra Komarovsky. Feldman and Brightman synthesize the contributions of family studies to Leighton's theory; Komarovsky illustrates a framework for studying family life, with examples from blue collar workers. The summary of seminar ideas on how to study family processes and mental illness are included as an introduction to these two chapters. At the end of this summary, Isidor Chein presents a list of dimensions of family solidarity.

Chapter 10 is devoted to the relationship between work settings and mental health. Two seminar sessions dealt with this important subject. Out of these two very fruitful discussions, a summary of the essential ideas was distilled. Also included is an extensive discussion of the important and, apparently, neglected subject of job-cultures, which are apparently of profound importance, especially if we wish to move beyond simple social class formulations.

Chapter 11 deals with several fundamental conceptual and methodological problems: How do you identify the personal community of urban residents? What is a community? How do you measure the impact of the "setting" on its inhabitants?

It should be emphasized that Chapters 7-11 provide a variety of alternate strategies for studying social processes and mental health in urban settings. If one studies the social units of residence, family, work, or behavioral settings, what conceptual and methodological problems are involved? Especially, if the wish is to implement the basic concepts of integration-disintegration in urban social systems, what conceptual and methodological problems ensue?

Finally, the reader should also be alerted to the diversity of the book's format. Summary papers are included in some cases. At other times, excerpts of the actual exchange of ideas are presented. The reader will find that these conversations contain summaries of the basic ideas in a sans serif face preceding each conversation. Consequently, the book can be read to obtain summaries of basic ideas presented, single commentary statements, and actual conversations. In this way, maximum use is made of the seminar proceedings, and much of the natural history of developing research questions is preserved.

Cosmos in the Gallup City Dump

ALEXANDER H. LEIGHTON, M.D.

The first time I saw Bronislow Malinowski was when he came to Baltimore to speak at the Henry Phipps Psychiatric Clinic of the Johns Hopkins Hospital. It was my duty to meet him, and thus it was that I first saw him, advancing along a platform at Union Station brandishing a tightly wrapped black umbrella and saying, "I hope you will pardon this symbol of British acculturation."

This moment, early in the morning of an autumn day in 1937, brought together three major experiences. The first was getting to know Malinowski himself, vital and volcanic. The second was acquaintance with the functional orientation toward human affairs he contributed to the thinking of his time. The third was encountering "acculturation," a word which up to that instant I had not heard. Because all of these were influential in the development of the Stirling County Study, I have chosen the meeting with Malinowski as the starting point of the present chapter. This is in response to the editor's request for something about the origin of the study, and I hope that both he and the reader will be tolerant of the personal flavor that ensues.

The reason for cultural anthropologist Malinowski's visit to a psychiatric clinic was both general and particular. The general reason was that culture-and-personality as a field of interest was to the fore in the decade prior to World War II, and psychiatry was one of the approaches to the development of personality theory. Influential in this aspect of personality theory were the driving curiosity and creative thinking of such minds as George Herbert Mcade, W. 1. Thomas, Edward Sapir, Ruth Benedict, Margaret Mead, Ralph Linton, Clyde Kluckhohn, Morris Opler, and, of course, Malinowski.

These names refer to social scientists. Interest was less widespread in psychiatry but did hold a place in the speculation of several leaders, notably Freud in Europe and Harry Stack Sullivan and Abraham Kardiner in the United States. Aside from psychoanalysts, Adolf Meyer, then chief of the Phipps Clinic, was perhaps most outstanding for his interest in personality and in the molding effects of culture.

The particular reason for Malinowski's visit was an invitation from Meyer, given at my suggestion. A resident in the Phipps Clinic, I had become curious about how nonpatients handle the various life crises and problems of human relations that seemed to give the Clinic's patients so much difficulty. This line of questioning was strongly encouraged by Meyer who entertained doubt about the prevailing view that the answer to all important problems of personality would be found exclusively in the infantile period. He thought that some weight must also be given to transactions in the patient's current life situation, and he spoke about the formation of "self-defeating habits and of healthy habits." "Habits" were considered something one learned from one's social environment. Perceptions, goals, and values were other aspects of personality that, for better or for worse, the individual selected unto himself from the range offered by the situational accidents of his life and the culture of his society. Meyer argued for studying the healthy as well as the unhealthy and for considering both in terms of interaction with their context, current as well as past.

To my questions as how to go about a systematic study of context, Malinowski answered: "You are talking about American culture. But you are too close to it to see it. Go study another culture first. Only thus will you have the perspective for seeing your own clearly." Then he added a German saying which was translated something like this: "The more you know about others, the more you know about yourself."

This view was reiterated by a number of social scientists, and turned into an opportunity by a fellowship from the Social Science Research Council in 1939-1940 [1] and by the tutoring and field guidance of Clyde Kluckhohn. Major help was also given by Ralph Linton and Abram Kardiner.

Although Meyer's view of personality was more operational and more oriented by what he called "common sense" than is psychoanalysis, it was nevertheless dynamic. That is to say, it regarded every individual as the product of growth and as an integrate of interacting psychological components such that each component made a contribution to the behavior of the whole. Therefore, any given pattern of behavior—whether disorder or healthy—was to be understood not only in terms of life history, but also in terms of its current role in the behavior of the totality that was the person. It was, in short, a functional orientation, although the word was not used, and it was parallel to Malinowski's view of culture and its component cultural patterns. Both conceptions were holistic and both stressed the contemporary significance of any given behavior as influencing and influenced by the totality. Malinowski's "functionalism" was therefore congenial as a bridge between personality process and socio-cultural process and led me to explore such ideas further through the writings of Radcliffe-Brown and Durkheim. Much later this was amplified by Robert Merton, Bertanlafney, and Parsons, and particularly through many long discussions with E. H. Spicer, W. F. Whyte, and D. C. Leighton.

One consequence of the functional orientation (with regard to both personality and culture) is the requirement that one set aside his values and look at human behavior analytically in terms of what works and

[1] Held jointly with D. C. Leighton

what fails to work, and in terms of causal relations. This does not, of course, mean any long-range abandonment of values, for one can still wish to heal the ailing or to make the cultural environment more humane. It does, however, challenge one to turn away from partisan viewpoints, to overcome many personal defence mechanisms, to achieve, in short, a cognitive rather than an affective approach to human affairs. It goes without question that this is extremely difficult, demanding long and continuous practice, and is never wholly mastered. Meyer believed that a large part of psychiatric training was concerned with developing this ability, and Malinowski had it in mind when he recommended that I begin the study of American culture with observation of a wholly different culture, one in which the observer would not be so emotionally involved.

In choosing a cultural group for the proposed studies, it was desirable to find a place that would be reachable within our resources and yet not "spoiled," not "too acculturated." Thus Malinowski's little joke that he, a Pole, had acquired the British umbrella and carried it to America, took on new meaning. Most of the world, I discovered, was steeped in aculturation, and in the end I had to accept compromise. A group of Navahos was chosen under the advice of Kluckhohn and an Eskimo village on the recommendation of Ralph Linton. Both of these groups had acquired many elements of Western culture, but each also had retained much its own way of life. They presented marked contrast with each other and with "America."

Equipped with Meyer's view of personality and my adaptation of his study methods, I began with the Navaho. The aim was to collect life histories and to make direct observations regarding the lives of selected individuals. After repeating the same procedure among the Eskimos and later in an American community, I intended to make a comparative analysis that would bring out the relationship of culture to the strengths and weaknesses of personality. My hope was that through actual field work I could go beyond the hitherto largely speculative contributions of psychiatrists to personality theory and throw some light on just how culture exerted its influence and with what result. I wanted to be able to say something on the basis of firsthand evidence regarding the mental health and mental illness implications of being Navaho, Eskimo, or American. These aims were guided by anthropological views regarding cultural determinism.

In reflecting on the Navaho life stories as they unfolded and in watching daily activities around the hogans, my attention was attracted by an apparent association between psychiatric disorder and situations of rapid acculturation. A closer look suggested that this was not so much acculturation as the failure of acculturation. The Navahos with symptoms of this kind were those who had lost some vital hold on the ways of "the people," but who had not acquired an alternative. They were neither Navaho nor "American," but people without a whole and coherent culture.

Such a point had previously been made by various writers, but it did not occupy the center of the stage at this time. Both anthropological and psychiatric theorists felt there was deeper insight to be gained through the comparative study of personalities in different cultures with especial emphasis on child-rearing practices. Thus, at the beginning, I was far more interested in the impact of what survived of Navaho culture rather than in the study of people on the margins. The matter, however, would not stay out of sight and was dramatized by the predicament of families who lived on the edge of the city of Gallup, under conditions that have since in other places come to be called the "septic fringe."

A paradigm was provided by those who squatted on the city dump. It seemed clear that personalities being formed in such culturally confused and depriving circumstances were heavily exposed to noxious influences—according to any psychodynamic theory from Freud to the common sense psychiatry of Adolf Meyer.

This realization spurred me into making speculative comparisons with nearby Zunis and Hopis; all at once it seemed that the differential influences on personality, which everyone was expecting to find in subtle hues through cultural studies, were present in blatant primary colors on the Gallup dump. However important basic cultural differences in language, ideation, and child-rearing practices might turn out to be, there seemed little doubt that the contrast between the conditions of Indians in any going cultural system—whether Navaho Mountain, Zuni Pueblo, or the Hopi Mesas—and those in a shattered cultural no-man's-land was far greater than anything that could be found among the Indian cultures. The notion kept recurring that for understanding social environment and personality process, and especially for understanding conditions affecting mental health, perhaps acculturation is the portal of entry rather than the cultural determinants of basic personality. The fact that acculturation was engulfing the world and that cultural islands were growing fewer year by year, gave a quality of insistence to the idea. But the thought was an uncomfortable one because I felt much more drawn to whole cultures than to their rags and bones.

The Eskimo study brought up the whole matter again. The way to the village led through Nome, where once more the noxious effects of living between two worlds and not being effectively in either seemed plainly evident. For most Indians and Eskimos, furthermore, it seemed that the only opening into Western culture was at its lowest socio-economic level, at the level where Western culture itself has its greatest malfunction and the least resources for meeting creative needs and providing a basis for human dignity. Whatever the reasons, symbolically, the gateway was on the town dump.

The village, located on St. Lawrence Island, was by contrast to the Eskimo group in Nome, an exceedingly well put together community. It was a self-contained, self-integrating, resourceful, and effective human social system whose members held their heads high and survived in the face of appalling physical odds. While far from being culturally pure, it was a synthesis rather than a collection of cultural incompatibilities. The outboard motor, the gun, a reindeer herd, and such foreign institutions as village council and cooperative store had become effectively interwoven with traditional values and practices in family life, hunting, and religion. Change was still in progress, of course, and gathering speed through school and mission, but in 1940 the villagers—or as they called themselves, "natives"—were maintaining control of their equilibrium.

They were, of course, a world away from the Navahos in terms of culture, and yet it seemed that in personality assets they and the culturally strong Navahos that I had seen on the Rain Plateau had more in common than either did with their counterparts on the septic fringes of Gallup and Nome. Thus, there came again the nagging thought that perhaps I should concentrate my effort on precisely what my enthusiasm for culture and personality was leading me to avoid—broken cultures rather than comparisons of the functionally effective.

Two subsequent experiences served to further develop the line of thought. World War II prevented an immediate beginning on the third part of the original project—personality studies in an "American" community. Instead I was projected into witnessing and studying the evacuation and incarceration of Japanese and Japanese-Americans from the Pacific Coast. This was a demonstration of instant social disorganization—followed later by incredible recovery. The complexity and far-reaching quality of the catastrophe as effecting every major and minor psychological dynamic of the personalities involved was as evident and certain as a nonexperimental and nonstatistical observation about life can be.

The second experience was assignment to study the military and home front morale of Japan. This was at first done at a distance through documentary sources, but culminated immediately after the war in a survey of Hiroshima where instant disintegration was again seen but in new proportions. In this I do not refer to the physical destruction and loss of life as such, but to their consequences for the survivors, for the remnants who had been part of the system that had once been called Hiroshima. In this setting all human history appeared reduced to the stark issue of man's struggle against chaos within himself.

Thus, the notion seemed ever more compelling that order in the environment, or at least the resources to create that order, was essential to the human psyche. Without this it seemed that man quickly becomes alien to himself and prone to the conditions he calls psychiatric disorder. It was doubtless a former and partial recognition of this fact that led to psychiatrists once being called alienists.

When the war ended and opportunity came once more to study personality process and sociocultural process, I reconceptualized these as systems within systems and as systems interlinked with systems. The originally projected plan for investigating an American community became the Stirling County Study. Tucked into this was still the idea of personality studies that would ultimately be compared with Eskimos and Navahos. This aspect, however, was now overlaid in my mind with the problems of order and disorder in societies and persons. To this was added the desire to deal in quantitative data wherever possible, a natural outgrowth of the earlier exploratory studies and of clarification regarding the kind of data needed. It was on account of this desire to speak definitively about "how many" and "how much" in comparative statements that the work took on an epidemiological cast. The development of the Stirling County Study itself is taken up in the next chapter.

As a concluding note here, it is of interest to observe that the meaning and significance of order, organization, and integration both psychologically and socially, have year by year intruded more on everyone's awareness. At the present moment there are many who are willing to regard these as the enemies of mankind and to feel that salvation lies in the destruction of all systems: economic, educational, governmental, and religious. This may be transition to something better, but one cannot help but query as to whether mankind can survive the transition. Certainly there is a body of evidence worthy of serious consideration that suggests that disintegration is lethal. The world could well destroy itself without nuclear war. Centrifugal forces of individualisms unbalanced by centripetal forces of organization could amount to just that: utter fragmentation and destruction.

One is tempted to say of the "cosmos," but as we have come to use that word, it means more than the world. Perhaps this is rightly so. In its original Greek meaning it stood for neither world nor universe.

It meant order.

3

Some Notes on Objectives

JANE M. MURPHY, Ph.D.

Our purpose is to develop conceptual clarity about social processes that influence mental health and mental illness, especially in large urban areas. The following are some ideas on this topic. They are not intended to limit the scope of the seminar but to stimulate discussion by suggesting a few starting points. In essence they represent some of the preoccupations which led to the development of the Cornell Program in Social Psychiatry.

The program as a whole consists of two interlocking parts. One is concerned with the validity of concepts of psychiatric disorder used in survey work such as the Stirling and Midtown studies. The other part deals with the questions to be considered by this group, that is, the development of hypotheses and operational steps for testing the validity of social concepts pertinent to psychiatric disorder.

The main approach in the Stirling Study is the investigation of social integration and disintegration. In brief, "integration-disintegration" refers to a continuum of states, characteristic of social interaction systems, varying from functional effectiveness to ineffectiveness. In the Stirling Study we used "communities" as geographically localized interaction systems in which to investigate these processes. We hypothesized that if noxious social conditions were to exist long enough and with sufficient severity in a community, disintegration would occur. Conditions that might have this effect are: (a) major disasters, (b) widespread ill health, (c) extensive poverty, (d) cultural confusion, (e) marked secularization, (f) heavy migration, and (g) very rapid and pervasive cultural change. It was feasible in Stirling County to use the conditions of poverty, secularization, and cultural confusion taken in combination as indicators for identifying socially disintegrated communities. It was further hypothesized that the process of disintegration would be characterized by a number of symptomatic features: (a) high frequency of broken homes, (b) few and weak associations, (c) few and weak leaders, (d) few patterns of recreation, (e) high frequency of hostility, (f) high frequency of crime and delinquency, and (g) weak and fragmented networks of communication. From the viewpoint of theory, an important aspect of the disintegration idea is that it refers to an over-all pattern. This total pattern is more than any single discrete social condition such as poverty. If this kind of over-all state pertains in a social system, psychological stresses will be felt by the people who make up the interacting unit and these stresses lead in turn to psychiatric disorders.

In the Stirling study, it was found that the communities selected by the three identifying criteria did in fact exhibit the features symptomatic of disintegration and further, that a significant correlation was found between disintegration and prevalence of psychiatric symptoms.

With this as background, some of the areas of interest in formulating future work can be described.

(1) Can we develop research that will test the "construct validity" of integration-disintegration? In this exercise, can we improve the operational definition, clarify the concept, and develop pertinent theories? There are two orienting questions regarding the "construct validity" of the disintegration concept: (a) Does the concept refer to real social processes that can be objectively demonstrated? (b) Is disintegration a useful concept for assessing and predicting the character of social process relevant to psychiatric disorder?

(2) What, in more detail and in process terms, is the nature of the social phenomena to which our operational indicators of disintegration refer? Since a fundamental reason for interest in a concept such as disintegration is the desire to understand the effects of social processes and the interrelations of processes rather than isolated and segmented environmental factors, the longitudinal dimension is important. What can be learned by watching and describing disintegrative and integrative processes through time? Does a disintegrated environment become integrated when theoretically defined and objectively identified changes occur or are introduced? Can predictions be made on the basis of concepts and criteria and then tested by independent observations (analogous to "predictive validity" in the field of psychological test development)? Can, for example, the conditions be defined under which change will and will not produce disintegration in a social system?

(3) The concept and operational criteria of disintegration can be refined by comparisons in groups that differ from each other in cultural patterns. For example, family unity is one of the indicators of socio-cultural integration employed in the Stirling setting. This was also applied in our study of Yorubas in Nigeria, but inasmuch as the family structure there includes polygyny, the operational criteria for getting at the same underlying process had to be modified and adapted. Similar adjustment had to be made with regard to such indicators as leadership, the presence of formal and informal organizations, and economic self-sufficiency. Field trials of this type progressively delineate the concept to bring it closer to nature and sharpen the criteria that can be used in hypothesis building and hypothesis testing.

In addition to cultural contrast, similar advantages could be derived from comparison of communities that are much farther apart in the matter of integration and disintegration than in any study to date. In this way more objective and valid criteria might be singled out and tests of reliability and validity developed.

In terms of utilizing comparison of contrasting units as a way of exploring the validity of a social concept, the comparison of urban and rural groups is perhaps one of the most provocative resources open for immediate consideration by our study group.

(4) When one turns to an urban environment, the concept and indicators of disintegration must be adapted to an infinitely larger and more complex mass of interdependent processes. Up until this point in our studies we have always underscored the fact that integration-disintegration refers to the over-all pattern of functioning within an ecological system. The "community as a whole" has been an appropriate referent and unit of analysis. If we were to carry this aspect of the concept through its logical sequence in studying an urban environment, it would be necessary to focus on the "city as a whole." It is reasonable to suppose that social disintegration could occur so that it would affect a whole city (for example, the bombing of a city during war). The chief value of the "city as a whole" approach, however, would derive from investigating several cities in a comparative frame of reference in order to make and test predictions about differential prevalence of psychiatric disorders. It is not very practical to think of undertaking the massive research necessary to such rigorous consistency and more importantly, it is probable that there are interaction systems within a city that have more crucial and perduring significance for mental health. What are the types of interaction systems in an urban environment to which the integration-disintegration concept can be applied? Can they be isolated, and can investigation be carried out so that a valid comparison can be made with systems in a rural environment? Is the idea of "community," either in terms of geographic locales or conceptual variants of this prototype, helpful in studying integrative and disintegrative processes in a city?

A common method of subdividing city populations is by socio-economic class. It is well known that in previous urban studies, class has provided a way of separating noteworthy differences in the prevalence of disorder. The question now is, "Where do we go from here?" Can we move from the correlations with class to the uncovering of other relationships? Do the integration-disintegration concepts and methods offer any assistance in this? Can various systems of social interaction and networks of communication be identified within classes, or cutting across class lines, that can be analyzed on a continuum of integration-disintegration? Some of the examples of the systems in mind are: family, work place, circle of friends, religious group, recreational activities, and ethnic units.

(5) There is need for simpler and more quantifiable means of identifying disintegration. For instance, preliminary trial of Barker's "behavior settings" has indicated that this may be an approach worthy of further investigations. In the communities studied in Stirling, the number of settings has proved to be inversely proportional to disintegration as measured by other means. Can the quality as well as quantity of settings be incorporated into the indices of integration-disintegration in a city? Can the "settings" approach be tried out in a sufficiently large number of contrasting environments so that tests of reliability and validity can be run?

(6) Thus far we have dealt with the processes of integration-disintegration entirely at the level of analyzing whole social systems. This is distinguishable from the area of interest that is concerned with the interphase between an individual and those properties and processes of the social group of which he is part. What is it about disintegration that accounts for the high correlation that has been found with psychiatric disorder? What are the intervening factors between the global typology of an environment defined as disintegrated and the prevalence of psychiatric disorder? For example, a community *qua* community may display the characteristics of integration but not everybody will necessarily experience it as an integrated environment. What methods could be devised for sorting out and classifying individual variations in the experiencing of social processes so that significance for mental health will emerge?

(7) Some leads on the last point have come from work in Stirling and

among Yorubas and Eskimos, where our studies indicated that socio-cultural disintegration has a differential effect on men and women. In one community one sex will appear the more affected, while the reverse will be the case in another community. Inasmuch as this seems to be a matter of the way in which various roles are related to the processes of a particular social system, one may ask if major role categories can be defined (for example, age and occupation positions as well as sex) in order to see which are particularly susceptible to this kind of variability. What elaborations would be necessary for developing a role classification for an urban area?

(8) Urban social systems and the roles they comprehend usually concern only a portion of the lives of the people who compose them. Any one person or category of persons may have his life projected through several of these systems and roles. Thus the relationship between systems as well as the character of any one system becomes a matter of importance in developing and testing theories of the effects of socio-cultural environment on mental health. Is it possible to construct a formula that would properly proportion such aspects as: the number of systems in which an individual has social identity (the isolate versus the joiner); the saliency of some interacting systems over others; the congruence or dissonance between systems; the quality of systems in terms of level of integration-disintegration; and the significance of particular role positions in different systems?

(9) What is the relationship of socio-cultural integration to mental health and psychiatric disorder? As a framework for hypothesis building we suggest that while *dis*integration is damaging to mental health, *in*tegration is not necessarily beneficial. It is a necessary but not sufficient condition for mental health. For example, Sparta was well integrated but it seems unlikely that it was a mentally healthy place for the Helots who made up a large part of the population. This suggests the studying of different patterns of integration to discover if some types are more associated with psychiatric health than others. Through

this means it might be possible to approach the question, "What causes mental health?"

4

Psychiatric Disorder and Social Environment

An Outline for a Frame of Reference [1]

ALEXANDER H. LEIGHTON, M.D.

My aim in this article is to suggest a conceptual bridge whereby certain aspects of personality, viewed as a process, and certain aspects of society, viewed as a process, may be related to one another. The work took origin in the need for a frame of reference in a particular research task (The Stirling County Study) concerned with the effects of sociocultural factors on the prevalence of psychiatric disorder.

A frame of reference is considered desirable (1) as a means of indicating the range of phenomena to be considered; (2) as a means of indicating the range of different relations that may exist among them, and (3) to serve as a base from which to develop operational hypotheses and procedures.

A conceptual bridge is considered worthy of attention because, despite the unity of the phenomenon, man, the tools, both methodological and theoretical, for depicting and predicting individual behavior are different from those which serve the same purpose with

[1] From Bergen, Bernard J. & Claudewell, F. Thomas (Eds.) *Issues and problems in social psychiatry*. 1967, Chap. 8. Courtesy of Charles C Thomas, Publisher, Springfield, Illinois, with permission of the publisher, editors, and the author.

regard to societies. These differences lie in vocabularies and in contrasting levels and kinds of abstraction. Pathways must be found among these if one is to understand how social and cultural factors affect the ideas, feelings, unconscious motives, spontaneity, defenses, and other aspects of personality related to mental health. In swinging the point of one's attention back and forth between such concepts as cultural holism and personality holism, or between the function of a cultural pattern and the function of a psychiatric symptom, or between sociocultural organization and personality organization, there is need for some scaffolding of ideas by which interconnections may be traced.

THE AIMS OF THE STIRLING COUNTY STUDY [2]

The general purpose of investigating the influence of sociocultural

[2] The Stirling County Study has been conducted within the Department of Psychiatry, Cornell Medical College and the Departments of Sociology and Anthropology, College of Arts and Sciences, Cornell University. Financial support, for varying amounts of time, was provided by the Carnegie Corporation of New York, the Ford Foundation, the Milbank Memorial Fund, the National Institute of Mental Health, and from Dominion Provincial Mental Health Grants in Canada. These institutions are not, of course, owners, authors or proprietors of this report and are not to be understood as approving, by virtue of their grants, any of the statements of views expressed herein.
The author wishes to express particular thanks to the following: Urie Bronfenbrenner, John S. Harding, Dorothea C. Leighton, Charles C. Hughes, Jane M. Murphy, Marc-Adelard Tremblay, Robert N. Rapoport, and Robin M. Williams, Jr., all of whom played important parts in developing the ideas expressed in this paper.
A complete report of the Stirling County Study may be found in:
(a) Leighton, A. *My name is legion.* New York, Basic Books, 1959.
(b) Hughes, Charles C., Tremblay, Marc-Adelard, Rapoport, Robert N., & Leighton, Alexander H. *People of cove and woodlot.* Communities from the Viewpoint of Social Psychiatry (Volume II. The Stirling County Study of Psychiatric Disorder and Sociocultural Environment). New York: Basic Books, 1960.
(c) Leighton, Dorothea C., Harding, John S., Macklin, David B., Mac-Millan, Allister M., & Leighton, Alexander H. *The character of danger.* Psychiatric Symptoms in Selected Communities (Volume III. The Stirling County Study of Psychiatric Disorder and Sociocultural Environment). New York: Basic Books, 1963.

factors on psychiatric disorders has necessitated three major conceptual steps: (1) clarification of what shall be meant by psychiatric disorder and the development of working definitions which make sense both in clinical terms and in terms of field procedures for classification and counting; (2) clarification of what shall be meant by benign and noxious social factors from the point of view of mental health, and the development of working definitions which make sense in terms of the nature of social processes and in terms of field procedures for classification and measurement, and (3) the development of an analytical framework whereby the distribution of psychiatric disorders can be examined in relation to social factors so as to support, modify, or reject hypotheses and lead to the development of theory.

These broad considerations have been translated into an on-going program composed of five major operations that have been carried out to varying extent. The first consists in the assessment of the distribution of psychiatric disorder by means of a semi-clinical type of appraisal. In this, information gathered by field interviewers on a probability sample of a given population is evaluated by a panel of psychiatrists. The aim is to estimate the prevalence of psychiatric disorder regardless of whether the individuals in the sample have had treatment or not.

A second line of endeavor is the assessment of the distribution of psychiatric disorder by means of a psychological screening device. Here the same probability sample is used, and the aim as before is to approach a true prevalence study, but the method of rating is different; the results of answers to a much more limited questionnaire are scored according to statistically determined patterns of response known to be characteristic of groups suffering from psychiatric disorders.

A third operation consists in a systematic identification and specification of certain social complexes as healthy, unhealthy, and intermediate in their influence on the presence of psychiatric disorder. This means, in effect, predicting on the basis of anthropological and sociological data, which groups in a population are high and which low in frequency of psychiatric disorders. The work involves extensive use of both qualitative and quantitative methods.

The fourth operation, so far less well developed than the others, is concerned with an intensive study of both ill and well persons as a means of hypothesis construction. Such hypotheses are brought to bear on both the design of the research and on the interpretation of the resulting correlations between sociocultural processes and psychiatric disorder.

Finally, some experimentation in preventive psychiatry is being conducted in an effort to put to use returns from the basic research. This constitutes a major opportunity for checking hypotheses as well as for bringing about some practical benefits [3].

The frame of reference was developed as a guide for making and relating these multiple observations, and is here presented in a condensed outline. It is hoped that it may have some general interest, not only for those active in research of a like nature, but also for those more broadly concerned with the relationships of individual and group processes.

STRIVING AND INTERFERENCE—TWO FUNDAMENTAL ASSUMPTIONS

Inasmuch as the intent of this paper is to bring together and relate theories one to the other, it is much more concerned with the well established than with the new. My attempt is to outline as accurately as possible the main aspects of the phenomenon with which we deal—the relationship of sociocultural factors to psychiatric disorder. But since this phenomenon is imperfectly known, the outline is compounded of

[3] Leighton, Alexander H. Poverty and social change, *Scientific America*, 1965, *212* (No. 5), 21.

fact, accepted theory, assumption and speculation, and is consequently a tentative orientation.

An effort to sketch salient features demands not only abridgment and generalization but also translation into one comparable set of terms. For these reasons, the reader is apt to find many familiar and even commonplace ideas turning up in unfamiliar shapes. Moreover, he is likely to find them unattended by some of the specific qualities which give them greatest meaning in the theoretical system which he believes most accords with the nature of psychodynamics. Thus, one of the first observations presented—namely, that human beings exist in a state of striving—may seem to lack essential content to those who feel that libido, anxiety, aggression, or dominance is the primary motive. What is being sought here, however, is precisely the common characteristic in all these, shorn of the attributes which would limit it to one or another theoretical system. This is clearly a reversal of the customary practice employed when one is discussing several theories—the practice of giving emphasis to the distinctive.

As a starting point, let me note two fundamental assumptions which, in one form or another, are to be found in almost all theories of dynamic psychiatry: *A given personality exists more or less continuously throughout life in the act of striving* [4]*; and interference with that striving has consequences which often lead to psychiatric disorder.*

The assumption that interference with striving may lead to psychiatric disorder, however, does not imply that every kind of disorder has an equal chance of appearing. The words *psychiatric disorder* refer to various classes of phenomena which are traditionally grouped together in textbooks, although many are in fact very different

---

[4] "Striving" is intended to include the negative as well as the positive aspects: escape is encompassed just as much as the notion of pursuit. Hence, the child's desire to be loved by his mother can also be expressed as his desire to avoid her rejection.

in fundamental nature. Compare, for instance, psychosis and anxiety reaction [5].

A problem encountered here is that although one can be sure of different kinds of psychiatric disorder, satisfactory criteria for their identification and ordering in relation to each other have not been developed. For the present, designations based on a mixture of behavioral and etiological considerations must be used, designations which sometimes reflect and sometimes have little relationship to the fundamental nature of the phenomena. As a result of this situation, one can speak in general with some confidence of a number of etiological processes or antecedents, but one cannot always be sure of their presence, absence, or admixture in speaking of a particular case or type of case. Interference with striving is one such antecedent. Others are heredity, physical trauma, toxicity, and malnutrition. Since these antecedents are not mutually exclusive, but can occur in the same person with a cumulative effect on each other, the obstacles to setting up distinctive classes based on them is apparent.

There is, however, the possibility of predominance of etiological process, and of consequences that are characteristic of that predominance. In delirium, for example, we have a fairly characteristic pattern appearing as a result of toxicity. Some kinds of mental deficiency are apparently a consequence of heredity. In both instances, however, the possibility that other antecedents may also play a role cannot be excluded.

With this background, a further assumption may now be stated regarding the kinds of psychiatric disorder expected to follow interference with striving. I would like to suggest that interference-with-striving is most relevant to the psychoneurotic disorders, to the

[5] In general terms, one may say that psychiatric disorder means *abnormality*. However, despite the statistical standard implied in the latter word, the concept of abnormal also embraces the notion of malfunction as compared to some ideal state of functioning, a state which may not be statistically normal at all in a given population.

transient situational personality disorders and to the psychophysiologic disorders; that it is least relevant to disorders caused by or associated with impairment of brain tissue function and mental deficiency; and that, in a third group—the psychotic disorders and personality disorders—it is still of major importance, but that other equally important factors may also be at work, such as hereditary predisposition or the effects of organic agents (trauma and toxicity) [6].

STRIVING AS A FUNDAMENTAL CHARACTERISTIC OF PSYCHICAL LIFE

The act of striving implies an object [7]. Common observation makes it clear that each human being pursues in the course of his life many objects, some of which he regards with strong attachment and others with only mild interest. It is also evident that individuals often differ from each other markedly in the kinds of object they emphasize and that cultural groups, too, may be in sharp contrast in this respect.

Dynamic psychiatry recognizes the multiplicity of objects and the varying degrees of attachment people have to them, and asserts that these objects are means to an end. There are, however, different theories as to the nature of this *end* and the processes involved in its attainment and maintenance. This is, indeed, very close to the core of the matter so far as differences and dispute in psychiatric theory are concerned.

Important as the areas of dispute are, particularly since they may help generate new discoveries, it is also important to keep in sight that there are ideas shared by most, if not every school of thought. For example, nearly every one of them incorporates the idea that there is an optimal

[6] The clinical terms employed are those suggested in the American Psychiatric Association's *Diagnostic and Statistical Manual, Mental Disorders*, 1952.

[7] By dictionary definition, an object is "... that of which the mind by any of its activities takes cognizance, whether a thing external in space or a conception formed by the mind itself...." *(Webster's New International Dictionary.)*

psychological condition and that many kinds of object striving are basically concerned with its achievement or maintenance. This may be phrased as absence of anxiety, the gratification of instincts, the reduction of tension, and in many other terms. But whatever the content of a specific theory, all postulate a process that intervenes between life experiences and the development of psychiatric disorder. In order to emphasize this pivotal concept and at the same time avoid the particulars of any one theory, the name *essential psychical condition* will be used [8].

[8] The fact that the illustrations given above are negative, reflects much psychiatric theory. For example, Freud thought of the reduction of excitation, Horney and Sullivan emphasized escape from anxiety, Adler spoke of overcoming feelings of inferiority, and Fromm of decreasing the inhibitors of spontaneity.
There are some, however, who have emphasized the optimal state as having the positive component which is also included in the notion of the essential psychical condition. Taking "tension" to illustrate the point, I would say that the optimal state is not the absence of tension, but some degree that is intermediate between too little and too much. This is quite different from Sullivan's "euphoria" as a state of "tensionless bliss."
In broad terms I conceive the personality system as sensation seeking, as striving to function and to exercise its capabilities and find expression for many of its potentialities. Such a tendency is part of a general impulsion to look for experience that has its basis in the genes of the organism. Meyer had this kind of thing in mind when he spoke of spontaneity; existential psychiatrists give emphasis to it; so did McDougall when he pointed to dynamic striving as a basic characteristic of the personality system. Murray stresses the significance of "zest" and the "need for activity," and, with Kluckhohn, he has formulated the concept of "proaction" in contrast to "reaction." Similar orientations emphasizing the self-actualizing of personality have been presented by Maslow, Goldstein, and Rogers. See: May, Rollo; Angel, Ernest; & Ellenberger, Henri F. (Eds.) *Existence, a new dimension in psychiatry and psychology*. New York: Basic Books, 1958. McDougall, William *An introduction to social psychology*. London: Methuen, 1936, Pp. 304-10. Murray, Henry A. *Explorations in personality*. New York, Oxford University Press, 1938, Pp. 129-134. Murray, Henry A., & Kluckhohn, Clyde A conception of personality, in *Personality in nature, society, and culture*. New York: Knopf, 1953, Pp. 10 and 36. Maslow, A. H. *Motivation and Personality*. New York: Harper, 1954. Goldstein, Kurt *The organism*. New York: American Book, 1939. Rogers, Carl A theory of personality and behavior, in *Client-centered therapy*. New York: Houghton Mifflin, 1951, Pp. 481-533.
Olds has reported experimental work in which rats are seen to seek cerebral excitation by means of electric shocks. He feels that these studies call in question all theories that base motivation primarily on tension reduction or similar process. See: Olds, J. Self-stimulation of the brain. *Science*, 1958, *127*, No. 3294, 315.

This *condition* is, to repeat, conceived as a process, not as something static. It is perpetually being lost and recovered, and so may be imagined as constituting fluctuations about a point that moves along the course of life, maintained only through constant activity on the part of the personality system. The factors which influence it arise both in the environment and within the personality. It has, therefore, considerably different qualities at different periods of life, e.g., adolescence, the middle years, old age.

Before going on to a discussion of the relationship of the essential psychical condition to psychiatric disorder, a few observations should be made about the concept of personality. I give particular emphasis to *sentiments* (despite the old-fashioned connotations of the word) and *symbols,* because these abstractions offer a convenient bridge for conceptualizing relations between a given individual and the collectivity of individuals who make up his social environment.

All forms of dynamic psychiatry agree in regarding personality as an integrate unit and psychiatric disorder as a condition of malintegration. The details of these assumptions, however, have been developed in a variety of ways and with various emphases by different schools of thought. One such variant conceives personality to be an integrate unit, or pattern, made up of many functioning, interdependent subpatterns, only some of which are directly evident to the person himself or to others. The subpatterns may be considered in terms of affect (moods and emotions), cognition (the processes of thought), instincts or drives (inborn urges such as those connected with food and sex)—or in terms of various combinations of these tendencies, blended with the results of experience and learning, to form interdependent patterns, both active and potential. *Potential* implies that patterns may be stored away, yet remain available for action in response to certain kinds of situations.

The notion of sentiments is relevant to this emphasis. For the purposes of the present frame of reference, sentiments may be described as ideas charged with affect and exhibiting a tendency to recur. They are a union of affective, cognitive, and "instinctive" processes shaped in the course of experience and are represented by symbols [9]. The expression "represented by symbols" is intended to convey the idea that words, visual images, and other similar patterns can stand for sentiments both in the processes of mentation and in communication with other persons. These symbols are obviously learned in the course of development, as are the sentiments for which they stand, and they play a fundamental part in the integration of personality through organizing the affective, cognitive, and conative processes into some kind of harmonious interrelationship. In the mental processes, these symbols operate in such a way as to enable the personality to deal with past, present, and future. Much of this goes on in conscious awareness, but it also takes place below the level of consciousness. Although I assume that sentiments are formed in consciousness as a result of perceived feelings and experiences, I also think they may afterward be laid away at a level from which, though it is difficult to recall them, they continue to exert an influence on the person's perception of, and receptivity to, the ever-unfolding edge of new experience.

Personality, then, may be conceived of as an integrate unit of sentiments; the maintenance of that unit is a dynamic process in which integration is constantly being torn down and built up as a result of changes originating within the person (e.g., puberty) and changes originating in the environment of interpersonal experience; symbols standing for sentiments play a major part in this dynamic process, both in mentation and in communication with the other personalities that make up the social environment.

In relation to this concept, a psychiatric disorder in a given person is seen as disturbed integration of his sentiment system, and the symptoms used in diagnosing various clinical entities are largely the

[9] For a fuller discussion of this topic, see Leighton, A. *op. cit.*, 1959, Chapter VII and Appendix A.

behavioral manifestations of this disturbance. Both integration and disintegration (or malintegration), it must be added, are relative. Thus it may be anticipated that in real life neither the completely integrated nor the completed disintegrated personality will be found. Furthermore, it may be assumed that any one personality in the course of a lifetime will move back and forth a good deal between more integration and less integration.

With this discussion in hand, we may now reconsider the two fundamental assumptions given earlier. The first of these is represented by a diagram in Figure 1 [10].

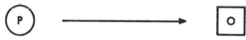

Figure 1. A fundamental characteristic of psychical life. P represents a person, the *arrow* indicates striving, and O stands for object. For any given P, the latter includes an enormous number of different particular objects which could be represented as O^1, O^2, O^3, etc.

Personality, that is the functioning of a person (P), would encompass the whole diagram. The relationship of the essential psychical condition to the psychical activity shown in the diagram is one of dependency. This may also be represented schematically as in Figure 1a.

The second assumption goes a step beyond these two diagrams and asserts that psychiatric disorder often (but not inevitably) appears as a

[10] The reader may note in this and subsequent diagrams similarities to the topological ideas of Kurt Lewin. Although the diagrams have not been derived specifically from a study of his work, it is likely that there has been some influence through conversations with Lewin and with several of his students. It is important to note, however, that the arrows in my diagrams do not correspond with Lewin's vectors, nor is personality to be equated with "life-space," although there is overlap in these concepts. Furthermore, my diagrams are not intended to be mathematical representations, but are merely illustrations of the type he described as holding "only in so far as the analogy holds," i.e., really only as long as it is convenient. As soon as consequences ensue which do not agree with the real facts, one evades the difficulty by asserting that it is after all only a model or an illustration. One says, "A comparison is not an equation." See: Lewin, Kurt *Principles of topological psychology* (Heider, Fritz and Grace, transl.). New York: McGraw-Hill, 1936, p. 79.

result of interference with the striving represented in the arrow. Let us set the disorder part of this aside for the time being, and examine this idea of interference in relation to the essential psychical condition.

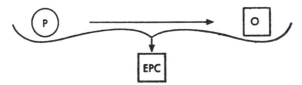

Figure 1a. The relationship of striving to essential psychical condition. Here P and O have the same meaning as in Figure 1, while EPC stands for essential psychical condition.

The objects in the sentiment system of any given personality are not all of equal functional importance to that personality. Some are peripheral to the essential psychical condition, whereas others matter a great deal to its maintenance. Of the latter, some are interchangeable objects—that is, can be replaced if removed from an expectation of achievement, but others are more unique in their relationship to the process. Overlooking for the moment the question of what kinds of objects fall in these various categories, it may be concluded that interference is significant when it intercepts objects that are important with regard to the essential psychical condition and that cannot easily be substituted. Furthermore, inasmuch as the essential psychical condition is always in a state of being lost and regained, the interference—to be dangerous for the system—must be drastic, must be of such magnitude, quality, or duration as to constitute a displacement far beyond the common fluctuations of the system and to tax severely the restorative capabilities.

Pervading all these considerations is the fact that the disturbing effects of an intereference in relation to a given personality depends on perception and expectation. Interference may not be "real" as strictly objective other persons might define it; the indispensable quality is that the person (P) perceive it as such. Perception and quality of anticipation in turn are determined by the sentiments the person brings to an event or series of events. Hence, an instance of interference with object striving consists in some kind of coming together within the personality of sentiments that are affectively and/or cognitively incompatible: "I need X, but I fear I cannot have X," "I want X, but I ought not to want X," "I do not want X, but I ought to want X," and so on.

The sentiment system may be considered as existing in the cross-section of the moment, derived from the past and looking to the future. It is in this sense the future exerts a powerful influence on the essential psychical condition of the present. Striving in relation to an approaching need may thus be crucial for the maintenance of the essential psychical condition and hence for the functioning of the person.

Discussion of perception raises the question of unconscious process. In this paper I am limiting "object" to entities which a given personality has readily available to awareness. Hence, sentiments are by definition conscious, or available without much difficulty to consciousness. What may be unconscious is a part of the chain of connections relating an object to the essential psychical condition. That is, in consciously striving for an object a person is generally not aware of all the functions which this object (as a representation in the mind) and this striving are playing in the integration and equilibrium of his personality.

In pointing to unconscious urges as underlying object striving the way is opened for speaking about "unconscious objects." Thus a man may consciously drink to excess because of an unconscious wish to destroy himself, which, in turn, may arise from an unconscious desire for revenge on someone by means of suicide. It would be possible to speak of the alcohol, the suicide, and the target of the revenge all as objects. In the present context, however, the word *object* is reserved for the conscious goals in such a web of interconnected factors, and the other items are designated as *motives*. This usage is arbitrary of course, but it emphasizes a distinction of importance.

ESSENTIAL STRIVING SENTIMENTS

It has been noted that the objects for which people strive are enormous in number and diversity and this makes it necessary to consider some ways of organizing them into categories for the sake of conceptual management.

The criterion for building categories relevant to our purposes here is the saliency of objects with regard to the essential psychical condition. Unfortunately, there is no way of ascertaining this directly, but some indications can be had from clinical psychiatry. One may ask what kinds of objects appear in those interferences with striving that are important in the disorders of patients. Such objects must by definition be among those closely tied to the maintenance of the essential psychical condition. There may, of course, be other objects intimately connected with the essential psychical condition which never come to clinical attention because of no interference, successful compensation, or other reasons. At the least, however, it can be said that the objects which do emerge in clinical work are a partial list of those important to the essential psychical condition.

With this as a guide, a list of essential striving sentiments according to object types has been compiled [11]. Although the number is ten, it is

[11] The main basis for this compilation is experience and theory in psychiatry. I am particularly indebted to Urie Bronfenbrenner for a review he made about the time the frame of reference was being developed. See Bronfenbrenner, Urie Towards an integrated theory of personality, in Blake, Robert R., & Ramsey, Glenn V. (Eds.) *Perception, an approach to personality*. New York: Ronald, 1951.
Impressions have been drawn in addition from psychology, social psychology, and cultural anthropology, though it would be hard to give specific references. Other influences stem from personal experience, not only in clinical psychiatry, but also in morale assessment and in conducting personality studies of non-patients in several cultures and under a number of different kinds of stressful circumstances. See: Leighton, Alexander H. *The governing of men*. Princeton: Princeton University Press, 1946 and *Human relations in a changing world*. New York: Dutton, 1949.

apparent that this total is most arbitrary. Given the complexity and intertwined character of human patterns of behavior, the number could be compressed or expanded according to purpose. The effort here has been to make a list as short as is compatible with the aim of using the frame of reference for a guide in research and hence ultimately mapping working categories.

Inasmuch as the types of objects have relevance only as they are part of sentiments closely connected to achievement and maintenance of the essential psychical condition, the categories will be called *essential striving sentiments*. It is to be recognized that each is actually a cluster of many topically related sentiments.

1. Physical security.
2. Sexual satisfaction.
3. The expression of hostility [12].
4. The expression of love.
5. The securing of love [13].
6. The securing of recognition [14].
7. The expression of spontaneity (called variously positive force, creativity, volition) [15].

[12] As conceived here, it is not necessary that hostility be always expressed in a socially or personally destructive manner. The idea is rather that hostility has to be expressed through the instrumentality of some patterns of behavior, if the essential psychical state is to be maintained. It is the type of pattern the person adopts that determines whether there will be socially and personally constructive or destructive consequences.

[13] The question might be raised whether this item should not be combined with Item 4 (the expression of love). They are kept separate here because it is thought that often in life situations the striving toward one may be satisfactory when the striving toward the other may encounter serious interference. For the same reason, Item 2 (sexual satisfaction) is not combined with Items 4 and 5.

[14] This too might be combined with Items 4 and 5. But, since the specific object pursued in this connection may differ very radically from those connected with love, it was thought better to list it separately. Recognition may be concerned with status and prestige and have relatively little to do with warm human feeling.

[15] The essence of the positive force is an urge to action over and above response to external stimulation.

8. Orientation in terms of one's place in society and the places of others.

9. The securing and maintaining of membership in a definite human group [16].

10. A sense of belonging to a moral order and being right in what one does (being in and of a system of values).

It is not necessary to assume that all these kinds of essential striving sentiments are equally significant in the achievement and maintenance of the essential psychical condition. The list is intended as a collection of probabilities, as a statement of major striving patterns in human behavior. It is likely that their relative importance varies at different periods in the course of life.

TYPES OF INTERFERENCE WITH STRIVING

Situations arising in the environment may interfere with essential striving sentiments. Figure 2 represents such conditions.

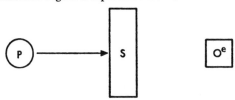

Figure 2. Interferences due to intervening circumstance. S is a situation arising in the sociocultural environment that cuts through one or more of the striving sentiments and bars the person from achievement, or the perception-anticipation of achievement, of the relevant object. P stands for person and O^e for objects in those striving sentiments which pertain most intimately to the essential psychical condition. Personality as the functioning of the person would again encompass the whole diagram.

[16] This may appear similar to Item 8. There is a distinction, however, in that Item 8 refers to a sense of orientation—knowing where one is in relation to others; Item 9 refers to the need for a sense of belonging. An isolated person could satisfy the conditions of Item 8 without satisfying the conditions of Item 9.

At the point in an individual's life story represented by this scheme, the personality is thought of as having been up to now adequate in its striving capabilities, and the types of specific objects for which it strives (the O^1, O^2, etc., which make up O^e) are thought to be appropriate in terms of the opportunities ordinarily available in the society and the culture. Loss of money or the threat of it might act as an interference through affecting the essential striving sentiments concerned with physical security, recognition and orientation in terms of one's place in society, and with maintaining membership in a definite human group. Another illustration is bereavement, which can operate in a similar manner through affecting sentiments related to giving and securing love, sexual satisfaction, and the expression of hostility. Rejection in love commonly touches on a number of the same kinds of sentiments as bereavement.

Recalling Figure 1a, the effect of such interferences on the essential psychical condition may also be diagramed, and this is shown in Figure 2a.

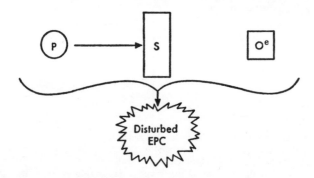

Figure 2a. The relationship of interference to essential psychical condition.

Here the meaning of P, S, and O^e are as in Figure 2. EPC stands for essential psychical condition, and the margins are jagged to indicate disturbance.

This same relationship of interference to essential psychical condition also obtains with regard to Figures 3 and 4, which follow, but it does not seem necessary to repeat the EPC diagram in each instance. The nature of the object incorporated in one or more of the essential striving sentiments may interfere or seem to interfere with their achievement. This is represented in Figure 3.

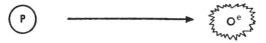

Figure 3. Interference due to the nature of the object. The irregular outline of O^e indicates defect in the object. Otherwise the functioning of the person and his pattern of striving are assumed to be adequate.

A man could, for instance, work over a period of years to qualify himself for a particular occupation from which he expected to gain physical security, recognition, orientation in society, membership in a human group, love, and other items relevant to the ten clusters of essential striving sentiments. If, however, by the time he has become qualified, a technological change has made obsolete the occupation for which he prepared, then one can say the object has become defective so far as its function in the essential striving sentiments is concerned and as a means toward the integration of his personality. By its very nature it prohibits fulfillment. Such a failure is due to changes in the society which it is conceivable have similarly affected many other persons preparing, or prepared, for the same way of earning a living.

Failure of an object to provide a necessary component in the functioning of a sentiment is but one of three primary difficulties of this general type. A second kind of defect is that in which a person strives for mutually incompatible objects. Thus, he may have an occupation which provides physical security but is low in recognition. The converse can also exist, as it often does with ministers and teachers. More dramatic, and possibly more dynamically significant, is the situation in which the objects of sexual satisfaction and love run counter to adequate fulfillment of most of the other essential patterns. Here the conflict with the need to belong to a moral order and feel right in what one does may be particularly sharp. [17] .

The third type of defect which may stem from the nature of objects is the situation in which the objects available for incorporation in the essential striving sentiments are so multiple, so ill-defined, or so few that it is difficult for the personality to develop a consistent or stable set. Thus, no one road to physical security, love, recognition, membership in a human group, or place in a moral order is clear enough to permit the establishment of sentiments that are functional in the personality system. One finds himself surrounded by vague, shifting objects toward which he is unable to develop strong attachment. Everything appears like everything else, every value has an equal opposite, and nothing provides a reliable opportunity for fulfilling the patterns upon which the essential psychical condition depends. This sort of thing happens not infrequently when a society is in transition from one culture to another.

What has been said thus far in discussing Figure 3 is over-schematized, and some word of qualification is in order. In the first place, the difference between Figures 2 and 3, although conceptually convenient, is largely a matter of definition. A second point is that Figure 3 may appear to equate object with person, that is, treat them as if they were

[17] The incompatibility of objects is not purely a matter of logical relationships. It is possible for the sentiment system of a personality to incorporate objects which are by rational standards in conflict or mutually exclusive without producing disturbance of the essential psychical condition. This occurs when the nature of the objects, the environmental situation, or the personality is such that the incompatibility reaches awareness only vaguely or not at all. This can be accidental, as when the sentiments containing opposed objects crop up at such different points in the weekly or monthly round of existence as to make the conflict difficult for most persons to perceive; or the lack of recognition can be more motivated as for instance when an inhibition of conflict-recognition serves to avoid disruption to the functioning of the sentiment system and hence the personality. See Leighton, A. *op cit.,* 1946, Pp. 228-292.

the same order of "thing." As mentioned earlier, however, objects may be things or they may be relationships. More than this, whether things or relationships, the objects are not so external to the person as the diagram suggests. Their existence for him (representation in his mind) is what counts, and this is a part of the functioning of his personality.

Most of the objects of striving sentiments which a person comes to incorporate in his personality have, however, been acquired from the sentiments which prevail in his family and in the society in which he grows and lives. Many of these were held by others and expressed by others before he was born, and in this sense the objects existed apart from him. In his life, he has found available a range of striving sentiments presented by the other people who are his social environment, and from these he has acquired and is acquiring his own particular collection. In this sense, then, one may speak of the social environment as providing effective or defective objects with reference to maintaining his essential psychical condition.

A defect in the functioning of a given personality may result in failure, or the perception-anticipation of failure, in one or more of the essential patterns of striving. This is shown schematically in Figure 4.

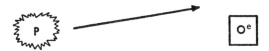

Figure 4. Interferences located primarily in the person. The irregular margins of P are intended to represent a deficiency in the function of a given person, while the direction of the *arrow* (missing the object O^e) is intended to indicate functional failure of relevant sentiments in the personality system.

Mental deficiency illustrates such a defect in personality. While this type of psychiatric disorder is not in its origin thought to be primarily consequent on interference-with-striving, it can be instrumental in the failure of one or more of the essential striving sentiments such as those pertaining to physical security, obtaining recognition, or orientation as to one's place in society, and thus lead to disturbance of the essential psychical condition. This in turn may lead to other symptoms of psychiatric disorder, over and above those inherent in mental deficiency.

It is probable that there are hereditary defects of affect somewhat parallel to the cognitive defects of mental deficiency. An inborn tendency to excessive fear, for example, might produce inaction or exaggerated behavior so as to interfere seriously with the development and functioning of one or more of the essential sentiments. The same might be said for other kinds of emotions, for lability and instability of emotions, and for speed of responses. It may be noted, furthermore, that *too little* may be as damaging as *too much*; too little flexibility of emotions may also interfere with the development of the essential sentiments.

Thus it would come about that some personalities have not merely malfunctional essential striving sentiments, but lack some of the categories altogether [18]. It is conceivable, for instance, that a person might have little or no basic urges of a sexual character. Such a condition would be bound to affect the whole organization of his personality. He might be compared to one who is tone-deaf and has the problem of adjusting to a world of music and of people who are not tone-deaf, or one who is color-blind but must live among those who have sensitivities and enthusiasms for color.

Incapacities besides the absence or near absence of sexual interests may also occur. The ability to give and receive love might be such another example. Here it is almost certain that some kind of sociopathic behavior would result.

What I am saying, in effect, is that there can be some kinds of psychiatric disorders without antecedent disturbance of the essential psychical condition. When such disorders occur, however, they are apt

[18] This point, a significant one for the frame of reference, was drawn to my attention by Toshio Yatsuchiro.

to bring with them disturbance of the condition and hence lead to the development of further disorder and further symptoms. The kinds of defect represented in the diagram are not limited to those that are inborn. It is possible for defect to be acquired, at some point in life, and to act thenceforward in the same manner as one that is inborn. Brain damage is an obvious example, but acquisition can also take place at more subtle levels. Thus if an upset in the essential psychical condition leads to chronic malfunction of the personality (e.g., excessive suspiciousness) by any of the means to be discussed in the next section, this defect can then act in much the same way as brain damage, namely, cause interference with the formation and adequate functioning of one or more of the essential sentiments. Thus the process of symptom formation and symptom persistence can become circular, or spiral, cutting deeper and deeper, once set going by a particular set of circumstances. Pathology or malfunction of the circular and spiral types, based on misfiring adaptations, is exceedingly common in nature, in all sorts of different contexts from cell physiology to social processes.

Looking at interpersonal relations in terms of roles suggest still another manner whereby a defect in personality may occur. In this view personality is conceived as composed of roles derived from other people. The self is a composite or "internal community" made up of appraisals from the "significant others" encountered in the course of life. The functional capabilities of each personality are therefore profoundly influenced by the quality and quantity of these interpersonal experiences. In order to have an opportunity for optimal development, a personality must interact with a fair cross-section of people representing the normal range of roles. Damaging consequences may occur if the individual has limited opportunity in this regard, or if among the range of his significant associates there is a weighting with persons who themselves suffer from psychological disorder.

An only child, to take an extreme example, who lives most of his life before adulthood in a socially isolated family will be cut off from his age-mates and may, because of the deprivation in his interactions, fail to develop a repertoire of roles for dealing with his peers. This can be carried into later life and lead to emotional problems. A child in this position is also likely to find trouble in his relationships with authority figures because his experience with them has been largely limited to his parents and hence too restricted and too specialized. If, in addition to all the above, one or the other of the parents is himself peculiar, the child's likelihood of psychological malformation is correspondingly increased through the incorporation of these peculiarities as part of the role. Personalities which are defective because their role relations have been defective may therefore be expected to have difficulties in the development of some of their essential striving sentiments. These in turn lead to instability of the essential psychical conditions.

Life history, therefore, is relevant to Figure 4, since the diagram represents the person (P) at some point in the course of his arc and includes both inborn difficulties of personality and those acquired at an earlier time.

ESSENTIAL STRIVING SENTIMENTS AND SOCIOCULTURAL ENVIRONMENT

A restatement here of the points developed thus far may be useful. It has been postulated that there exists in every personality an essential psychical condition, the disturbance of which may lead to the appearance of psychiatric disorder. The essential psychical condition is said to depend on a number of essential striving sentiments which have been described in ten major categories. The disturbance of the striving is pictured as occurring under three primary conditions: interference by the sociocultural environment in the striving, defect in those objects upon which the essential striving sentiments are focused, and defect in the already existing personality.

In the course of presentation, distinctions and categorizations have been made for ease in conceptualization and analysis. In nature, however, boundaries are indistinct and overlapping. It would be rare, indeed, to find pure interference in striving, pure defect in object, or pure defect in personality in any given instance. It is supposed here that the three generally occur together, but the relative weight may vary a good deal from personality to personality, at different periods during life, and from one set of circumstances to another. Many pastries, in short, have the same ingredients, but because the proportions differ, and the way of cooking, the results also differ.

Some of the environmental influences that can be significant for the production of psychiatric disorder may now be expressed in terms of the essential striving sentiments. Sociocultural situations can be said to *foster* psychiatric illness if they *interfere* with the development and functioning of these sentiments, since the latter in turn affect the essential psychical condition.

The sense in which *interfere* is employed has already been discussed. The word *foster* is used to indicate a preparation of the ground for some kind of psychiatric disorder, but without the further assumption that such disorder necessarily follows. As noted previously and as will be elaborated later, the disturbance of the essential psychical condition can be resolved without the appearance of those patterns of behavior commonly regarded as illness.

The relationship of environment may be put in terms of propositions and these are shown in the appendix.

ALTERATION OF SENTIMENTS THROUGH THE SUBSTITUTION OF OBJECTS

I wish now to suggest that an upset of the essential psychical condition, once it has passed a certain threshold, is felt by the person as unpleasant. A variety of words are commonly employed to represent this feeling, such as "anxiety," "tension," and "depression." Whatever the technical language the central idea is widespread in clinical psychiatry and may be stated as an addition to the fundamental propositions: disturbance of the essential psychical condition gives rise to disagreeable feelings.

An objection can be made to this on the ground that in many instances of interest to psychiatry the process takes place at an unconscious level, and hence there are no conscious feelings. I would agree with this in part and accept that much of what is going on is in fact commonly outside the area of awareness. In particular, the *source* of the disagreeable feelings is not apt to be apparent to the person concerned. Furthermore, due to malfunctional adaptations to be discussed presently, the disagreeable feelings may be diminished and masked without an accompanying restoration of the essential psychical condition. On the other hand, it is my assumption that at some time, and in some form, disagreeable feelings are involved and their imminent return remains a factor of importance in the functioning of the personality system [19].

[19] There are both semantic and theoretical problems interlaced in this question. One could well say that all that comes through to consciousness is the threat of a disagreeable feeling, something that is pale by comparison to the discomfort the underlying "thing" would yield were it to become manifest. This still leaves, however, some awareness of the disagreeable as part of the process and that is all the proposition says.

The possibility remains that the whole could transpire at an unconscious level. Some psychiatrists would maintain this view and, indeed, insist that this is the really important part of the matter.

For the purposes of this frame of reference I do not find such a view necessary. It would be foolish, of course, in the present state of our knowledge to deny that it could be so. Some of the satisfied sociopaths one sees offer temptation for believing it. In general, however, the patients one observes clinically are not happy about their condition. On the contrary, they are as a rule deeply involved in a struggle with disagreeable feelings. Furthermore, in the epidemiological surveys of psychiatric disorder conducted in Stirling County and elsewhere the same characteristics of unhappiness have been found in most of those persons who have never sought or had psychiatric treatment, but who were nevertheless rated as having psychiatric symptoms to a significant degree.

Given the disagreeable feeling—or the prodromal feeling of its possible breakthrough to consciousness—the personality reacts in the direction of getting rid of it. One form of this consists in altering the focus of the relevant essential striving sentiment, namely, changing the specific object. If, for example, an essential striving sentiment concerned with physical security, love, or recognition meets with interference, the latter may often be eliminated by shifting to another object. The action may take the form of a job change, a new person to love, or an attempt to seek membership in a group where recognition can be obtained, and so on. The possible specific illustrations for all ten of the essential sentiment clusters are, of course, virtually endless.

Thus, substitution of objects to eliminate perceived or anticipated interference in essential sentiments, without altering the essential functions of the sentiment, may be regarded as the personality's first line of defense—as prevailing, continuous and on the whole successful in maintaining the essential psychical condition. It can be compared by way of analogy with man's ability to maintain his body upright while walking over uneven ground.

These points are worth emphasizing since in psychiatry we have had some tendency to overlook the resources of object substitution. This is perhaps because the problems of the patients we see draw attention to instances in which such substitution is ineffective and other processes are in evidence. It seems to me, however, that the matter is worthy of careful exploration, particularly with regard to defining successful psychological function and building concepts of mental health that encompass more than the absence of psychiatric disorder.

It is pertinent to note that a common characteristic of objects (with relation to the essential clusters of sentiments) often favors substitution. This is because a great many discrete and specific objects can be encompassed in any given cluster of sentiments, so that the blocking of one has little effect on the system as a whole, and hence on the essential psychical condition.

STEPS IN THE DEVELOPMENT OF PSYCHIATRIC DISORDER

A disturbed essential psychical condition can lead toward the emergence of a psychiatric disorder if object substitution is not successful and the interference with essential sentiments continues. Again, it may be noted that common relationships between objects and essential sentiments favor this state of affairs. Some objects are by their nature not readily replaceable for most personalities. In this class belong those which occupy a key position in serving several different clusters of essential sentiments. A partner in love, for example, may also bring physical security, recognition, and a place in a definite human group. Such multifunctional objects, with a crucial position in many essential sentiments, are of great significance in the maintenance of the essential psychical condition.

Other factors also deserve consideration, of course, besides the nature of the object, such as the already noted cognitive and affective capabilities. Thus, the overall organization of personality might incline the individual to a rigid focus on certain objects no matter how impossible of attainment.

At the opposite pole from rigidity is the state of too great fluidity. Here, again, it may be a question of the nature of the objects, the nature of the personality, or both. A person can keep shuffling the objects relevant to his essential sentiments at a rate that amounts to disintegration of the sentiment system, and hence to failure in the integration of cognition, affect, basic urges, and unconscious processes. In such a state there can be no maintenance of the essential psychical condition, nor the cohesiveness and consistency as a unit necessary for adaptation to environment.

Object substitution may also turn out malfunctional due to the nature of the replacement selected. This, of course, brings us to the considerations already discussed in connection with inadequate objects and the diagram presented in Figure 3, but it suggests one reason why people may select inadequate objects. It may be a desperate choice.

In sum, the substitution of objects works well as part of the everchanging process of a personality in its course through life. Malfunction can occur, however, from one or both of two main sources: defect with regard to objects available in the sociocultural environment, and defect, inborn or acquired, in the personality.

The latter point may seem an instance of circular thinking, since the purpose of the scheme is to explain at least in part the evolution of defect. What is meant, of course, is that characteristics of personality antecedent to a given disturbance of the essential psychical condition may handicap the personality in using object substitution as an adequate defense or means of restoration. Hence the reasoning is circular, or spiral, only in that it reflects a process, psychopathology, which has this characteristic. The antecedent defects may belong in any of the categories already discussed under the headings of heredity and life experience, both physiological and psychological. The latter are notable for their capacity to develop progressive malfunction in which each step leads to the next, cumulatively, toward ultimate major disaster. One is reminded of the sequences by which the erosion of land sometimes occurs. A wheelrut on a slope will start the water cutting, and, as it cuts, the slope becomes steeper and the erosive power of the water and its silt increases.

The primary type of defective object is one that fails to restore the essential psychical condition. This is particularly so if the object selected is such that it eliminates, reduces, or disguises the perception of disagreeable feeling without having sufficient constructive effect on the underlying factors. For example, discomfort may be mitigated or removed, at least temporarily, by such agents as alcohol and drugs. A given personality may thus form a sentiment with one of these substances as the object, and this sentiment may come to occupy a central position in the personality, much as if it were one of the essential sentiments. In effect, it is such a sentiment, but one which is self-defeating because the disturbed essential psychical condition continues. More than this, the persistent expression in action of the sentiment may lead to physical depletion and interpersonal difficulties which directly and indirectly further increase the disturbance of that condition.

Excitement by means of sex and adventure can be employed in a similar manner to fill consciousness and crowd out awareness of suffering. The fact that sex itself constitutes a focal point in one of the essential clusters of sentiments introduces no contradiction, because in the instance suggested it is not a matter of fulfillment and hence maintenance of the essential psychical condition, but of using sex to mask feelings while leaving a disturbed essential psychical condition untouched, or making it worse.

Various other psychological processes commonly present in personalities can also be employed to modify disagreeable feelings without an underlying constructive effect. A person can, for instance, turn to daydreams while disengaging himself from interaction with other people that disturb the dreams. Fantasied objects and fantasied achievement are thus substituted for real life objects and real life acts and by this means the disagreeable feelings are masked.

As one variant in this process, a person may strive to establish the blame on someone else and become absorbed in elaborating and maintaining this view. Another possibility is to blame his body and find relief in preoccupation with his health. This can be diffused as general ill health, or focused on some organ or system such as the digestive tract. It may also take the form of a difficulty in using an arm or a leg, or even a sensory system, as for instance vision.

Forgetting, that is direct removal from consciousness, is also a psychological device by means of which to escape disagreeable feelings; in particular, painful memories and painful anticipations may be eliminated. Relief may be obtained, too, by attributing the disagreeable feelings to causes which, though false, are controllable, or seem controllable, such as germs. In this case, hand-washing and other ritual practices may constitute objects and focal points in sentiment systems which bring a sense of satisfaction.

The beginning of a trend in any of these directions may well be within the limits of behavior generally considered normal. It may in some instances be of considerable functional significance in providing an immediate relief from the pressure of the disagreeable, and thus enabling the personality to gird itself for a solution of the long-range problem through finding adequate objects. Taking a drink to cheer up, or a sleeping pill to get a good night's rest in the midst of one's worries, may not, in themselves, be malfunctional.

In many instances, however, there is a progression. Clinical observation suggests the occurrence of a series of steps in which each facilitates its successor toward one or another among the disorder patterns recognized in psychiatry. Thus, the trends noted above may go on to a sociopathic condition such as alcoholism, sexual promiscuity, and delinquency; or a schizophrenic type of psychosis; or a paranoid state; or such psychoneuroses as hypochondriasis, hysteria, amnesia, and obsessive-compulsive disorders. Since these various adaptations generally fail in completely masking or removing from consciousness the disagreeable sensations, there is commonly evident some mixture of anxiety, tension, depression, bitterness, and anger.

These progressive steps toward the formation of disorder have been here described with adult life in mind. The principle they illustrate, however, applies equally well to the earlier years, even though the content of the patterns is different. For example, in childhood the disturbance of the essential psychical condition might be due to deprivation in a basic urge for mother love. Despite the fact that at this stage of its development the personality has limited resources and alternatives, compared to the potentiality of later years, it will nevertheless make vigorous effort to shed the disagreeable feeling and restore the essential psychical condition. This can take the form of object substitution with sister, brother, or aunt, and it may or may not, in the long run, prove functional. The child personality can also turn toward psychological satisfactions divorced from reality, that is through the overdevelopment of autistic escapes, as with a dog or a toy. Diversions can also play a role through food, sexual pleasures, and emotional outbursts such as temper tantrums; or, the environment may be manipulated through negativistic behavior, refusals to eat, and other devices in order to promote attention as a substitute for love. The ramifications and variations are well known, but the point here is that they can be summarized as disturbances of the essential psychical condition with malfunctional patterns of restoration. Furthermore, such occurrences in early childhood may be and perhaps usually are the initial steps in progressive, cumulative development of psychiatric disorder which does not appear as overt symptoms until the adult years [20].

It should be noted that, for the purposes of this article, there is no need to explain the existence of fear, hate, love, sexual desire, depression, elation, aggression, suspiciousness, emotionally distorted thinking, retreat into imagination, and other patterns commonly evident in persons suffering from psychiatric disorder. These nouns apply to combinations and configurations of cognition, affect, and basic urges that are components of all personalities and are instances of the subsystems or parts which go to make up the self-integrating unit.

[20] This view of progressive disorder formation with one step leading to the next is derived primarily from study under Adolf Meyer who was in turn influenced by William James's ideas regarding habit formation and personality. See: Meyer, Adolf Remarks on habit disorganizations in the essential deteriorations, and the relation of deterioration to the psychasthenic, neurasthenic, hysterical and other constitutions (Pp. 421-431), Fundamental conceptions of dementia praecox, (Pp. 432-437), The dynamic interpretation of dementia praecox, (Pp. 443-457), The problems of mental reaction types, mental causes and diseases, (Pp. 591-603), in *The collected papers of Adolf Meyer.* Vol. 2, *Psychiatry*; Eunice E. Winters (Ed.) Baltimore: Johns Hopkins Press, 1951; James, William *The principles of psychology,* New York: Holt, 1890.

The unit is, however, integrating and in people not suffering from psychiatric disorder these components participate in the integration. Disorder therefore consists in distortion and disproportion in the functioning of such parts, and this is where explanation is sought.

From this point of view it can be seen as plausible and almost self-evident that some of the initial steps outlined as methods of seeking quick relief from the disagreeable consequences of a disturbed essential psychical condition will be employed from time to time by most personalities. Which steps occur in a particular person will be a matter of heredity, physiological experience, and psychological experience. The critical issue is that some people continue far into the progressive spiral of psychiatric disorder, while others stop or pull back. A point of attack for research is in the degree to which sociocultural factors, mediated through psychological experience, can determine one rather than another outcome.

It remains to consider the psychophysiological disorders such as headache, nausea, indigestion, peptic ulcer, hypertension, and asthma. This category encompasses symptoms of an organic type which have psychological factors as a major element in their origin and maintenance. Many of these same symptoms also occur primarily on an organic basis. Even when the psychological factor is the chief influence, organic agents may also be significant contributors, as for instance house dust in some cases of asthma. The central idea, however, is that a disturbance of the essential psychical condition can extend to a disturbance in the equilibrium of the whole organism. This amounts to a stress and response-to-stress complex in which there are many physiological ramifications, including reactions to organic agents.

That physiological changes accompany emotional states is self-evident on the basis of everyday experience. We flush with joy and grow pale when frightened, to take as examples of two acts which involve changes not only in the blood vessels of the face, but in much more of the circulatory system, including the contents of the blood, together with widespread endocrine and autonomic activities. It seems probable, therefore, that a disturbance of the essential psychical condition would produce physiologic alterations of some kind.

Before leaving this topic, it is worth noting that in addition to conditions placed under the heading of psychophysiological, some of the disturbances considered organic brain disease may have major psychological components in their origin. This applies particularly to the early onset and rapid advance of senility and arteriosclerosis.

STEPS THAT AVOID PSYCHIATRIC DISORDER

The substitution of objects mentioned earlier in this article is the main process by which interference with striving is eliminated and the essential psychical condition restored without the appearance of behavior likely to be called psychiatric disorder. The disagreeable feelings are corrected at their psychic sources and no crippling spiral is begun through immediate but not ineffective relief. The person selects new objects and maintains his essential striving sentiments in a manner compatible with both the needs of the personality system and the realities (including values) of the environmental situation. Since such behavior is also in the long run rewarding due to the reduction of disagreeable feelings, there is repetition of the constructive pattern in a manner similar to that described for the development of pathological patterns.

Beyond this, it is possible that out of this action something more effective than the previous level of functioning may evolve. The magnitude of the disturbance and the characteristics of the situation may result in the mobilization of capabilities in the personality that had not hitherto been active. Hence superior integration or productivity on the part of the personality can emerge, and it may be noted parenthetically that both pathology and unusual abilities can have their roots in disturbance of the essential psychical condition.

With regard to the psychophysiological types of disorders, it is evident that a restoration of the essential psychical condition would produce a more optimal state of the dynamic equilibrium of the whole organism. Hence one would not expect the appearance or persistence of disturbance to the vascular, digestive, and other systems—at least so far as psychological factors are concerned.

For the sake of presentation, the malfunctional and functional or healthy trends that may flow from disturbances in the essential psychical condition have been discussed and presented in propositions (see appendix) as if they were mutually exclusive. It remains to be said that they can, and do, occur in the same personality at the same time.

This notion may cause some readers to wonder whether the essential psychical condition is supposed to be both present and not present at the same time; for, if constructive restoration occurs, there is presumably no disturbance and hence no disagreeable feelings to induce the destructive spiral; or, is more than one essential psychical condition being posited?

Although it is true that the words "essential psychical condition" stand for a multidimensional process that could be considered in plural terms, this is not the point of the combined proposition BC (see appendix). It seems more useful to emphasize restoration of the essential psychical condition as having qualities of degree and stability. Thus a constructive trend may be only partially successful, leaving still-considerable discomfort as a focal point for the more or less destructive types of immediate relief; or, conversely, the existence of the immediate types of relief may handicap rather than eliminate the more long-range processes.

Stability implies restoration that is continuously effective during a major period of life. Instead of this, however, the restoration can be interrupted frequently, thereby giving the more destructive patterns opportunity for coming into play. Hence a period of life may exhibit alternating constructive and destructive trends.

This view says more than the generalization that people are complex and contradictory. It also does more than indicate again that personality, as the functioning of a human unit, constitutes the integration of many trends, some of them divergent. Stating the coexistence and alternation of effective and crippling processes with regard to the restoration of the essential psychical condition suggests that health and illness, however defined, must be regarded as states which consist in a kind of algebraic sum of opposite process. Many combinations are possible, with marked qualitative differences between them. It is commonplace, of course, to visualize psychiatric disorder in a variety of categories. Less often is it suggested that there are also many different healthy patterns. This combined proposition points away from a unitary concept of health and toward the idea of numerous patterns of psychiatric wellness. It points to mental *healths,* rather than mental health [21].

THE INFLUENCE OF THE SOCIOCULTURAL ENVIRONMENT

The formulations of this frame of reference do not yield any succinct or key-to-lock type of explanation as to why some people develop psychiatric disorders and others do not, or why among those who do develop disorders, some have one pattern of illness while others have another. Rather, starting with heredity, they postulate a range of factors, each of which is capable of exerting some influence on the outcome of a disturbance to the essential psychial condition in a given personality. The designation of these factors helps toward answers by pointing up targets of inquiry. Since our focus of interest is the influence of the sociocultural environment, discussion here will be limited to that kind of factor.

Having considered how the sociocultural environment may play a part

[21] For a discussion of the idea of "mental healths" see Leighton, Alexander H., Clausen, John A., and Robert N. Wilson, (Eds.) *Explorations in social psychiatry.* New York: Basic Books, 1957, P. 403.

in the disturbance of the essential psychical condition, the concern now is with its effect, once such a disturbance has taken place. Even so, however, there is some overlap of topic, for what was said earlier about the kind of objects offered by the environment to the unfolding personality also applies when it comes to the substitution of objects. Depending on its patterning, the sociocultural environment can steer a personality toward the development of disorder or toward nondisorder. More than this, if the trend is toward disorder, the environment can exert an influence regarding which type of adaptation occurs and hence have a differential effect on the patterning of the disorder, including its most obvious symptoms. On the other hand, if the trend is away from disorder, the environment can equally well exert a selective effect on which of many possible patterns of functioning, or mental healths, is actually adopted.

Sociocultural factors can exert this type of selective effect, not only on the more purely psychological disorders but on the psychophysiological illnesses as well. Thus, reactions such as headache, nausea, palpitations, diarrhea, and many more may be heightened or diminished by prevailing sentiments both toward the symptoms and toward the person who exhibits them. Apprehension about and efforts to conceal nausea, for example, may increase the sense of discomfort and thus adversely affect the total equilibrium, with the result that nausea becomes vomiting. On the other hand, in a culture where headaches are a cause for loving concern, and even a little prestige as a mark of driving oneself hard and being a bit of a martyr, there is apt to be some encouragement toward their emphasis and prolongation.

Sociocultural environment may also exert an influence on psychiatric disorder through the presence or absence of therapeutic resources, and in cases where these are present, through their nature and effectiveness. Where resources are numerous and effective, one may expect a smaller load of morbidity as compared to a similar situation in which these facilities are lacking. In speaking of resources, I refer, of course, to the formal therapeutic systems such as hospitals, out-patient clinics, and private practitioners. There is also need to recognize the importance of other institutions such as schools, churches, welfare agencies, and police, and of informal resources in wise men and women who, whatever formal roles they occupy, constitute advisors, therapeutic listeners, and confidants for their friends, neighbors, and relatives. It seems likely that many communities which lack all formal psychiatric treatment and in which the very name psychiatry is little known and less understood may, nevertheless, have numerous indigenous and valuable resources of a therapeutic character.

It remains now to consider further the nature of the social environment and to seek a framework for classifying it in units that can be studied and compared in terms of the conditions which have been described as relevant to psychiatric disorder. The first point to be made is that societies exhibit patterned arrangements of repeated interactions of their constituent members and that this integration is concerned with the performance of certain functions which are necessary for the survival and welfare of the society.

The statement that societies have functions recalls the proposition that the human being exists more or less continuously in the act of striving. This could be expressed in such terms as: the human being is always more or less in the act of performing certain functions which are necessary for his survival and welfare. In a similar manner, the assumption about societies can be restated as: human societies exist more or less continuously in the act of striving. The similarity of these assumptions suggests that the patterns of social integration which concern the performance of social functions may also concern the essential striving sentiments that have been postulated for individuals.

The primary functions of a society have to do with satisfying such needs as the acquisition of food, shelter, and clothing, protection of health, maintenance of law and order, defense against enemies, the birth and training of children, the satisfaction of sexual and other emotional needs indicated in the essential patterns, the provision of care in old age, and the disposal of the dead. All societies perform these functions, although the manner in which they do so—that is to say, the specific patterns—may differ greatly.

For purposes of this frame of reference, the fundamental propositions regarding the nature of society may now be stated as follows: (1) Human societies perform functions upon which their survival and welfare depend. (2) These functions are carried out by means of integrative patterns.

If integration and function are related, it would seem probable that different societies with different patterns of organization, and different subgroups in the same society—as well as different roles and combinations of roles within the society—might have differential effects in fostering the emergence and development of psychiatric symptoms through differences in access provided individuals for the satisfaction of the essential striving sentiments. It would also seem likely that groups seriously lacking in integration would have a high level of interference with essential striving sentiments and hence be prone to psychiatric disorder. The investigation of the influence of social and cultural factors on mental health could, therefore, be approached through examining the distribution of psychiatric disorder in one or more of the following contexts: cross-cultural comparisons, cross-subgroup comparisons within a given society, comparative analysis of roles, and comparative study of integrated and disintegrated groups. Each of these will be discussed briefly.

When one speaks of comparing cultures, it is of course with a view to selecting two or more cultures that present marked contrast in their performance of their functions. In areas of human relations that involve values, it is sometimes hard to say that one culture is better or more effective than another, since this may be a matter of taste. But if one considers a primary function, such as the provision of food, it is possible to point out that some cultures have subsistence techniques that keep them well supplied, while others, despite potentially adequate resources, are unable to avoid famine. Similar contrasts can be made with regard to the capacity for achieving protection from disease, as revealed in comparing mortality rates and life expectancy.

These considerations suggest that cultures may also differ from each other in effectiveness in fostering or interfering with the individual's ability to satisfy his essential striving sentiments. Just as some cultures do better than others in matters related to physical security, so they may differ in matters related to love, sexual satisfaction, recognition, and all the other needs upon which the essential psychical condition depends. In saying this, I am not ignoring the possibility that the shared sentiments of the culture may so color the perceptions of these matters as to minimize the traumatic effect of interference with these essential striving sentiments. My assumption is that, while such toning down of the consequence of deprivation does exist within cultures, it is not infinite. The essential striving sentiments are assumed to be panhuman, and hence there are limits to the deprivation that can be tolerated.

A second avenue for approaching the relationship of environment to mental health is in the comparison of subgroups within a given society. These groups—classes, associations, religious groups, and so on—are composed of human beings who spend most of their lives within their group. Possibly, therefore, as in the case of cultures, the subgroups of a society may differ from each other in regard to how well they provide the incumbent individuals with opportunities for fulfilling their essential striving sentiments, and for avoiding symptom formation. It may be that certain classes, associations, or religious groups present the maximum of healthful opportunities, while others are pathogenic. In such terms, then, an epidemiological study in a society might offer information that would be illuminating both with regard to the functioning of the society and the functioning of individuals.

In addition to considering the major subgroups of a society, attention could also be given to a small unit—the role. A role may be described as an enduring pattern of action and interaction carried out by a person so as to perform some aspect of a social function. While always manifest through the behavior of an individual, a particular role may be occupied successively by a number of different individuals, as for instance the role of teacher. A role is that aspect of behavior exhibited in such a pattern which is more or less constant, regardless of who fills the position.

A society can be regarded as having a network of roles, filled by a succession of different individuals. This turnover in the role occupants is due not only to death and birth, but also to changes in activity that occur in the course of individual lives. In addition, there is the fact that each person fills many different roles and moves about from one to another as part of his daily, weekly, monthly, and yearly activities.

Roles exhibit a wide range of difference in the degree to which they expose a given person to conditions bearing upon failure or fulfillment of his essential striving sentiments. This indicates the possibility of analyzing roles in a manner similar to that suggested for cultures and for subdivisions of a society, and of using a role network as a screen upon which to project an epidemiological study of psychiatric disorder. The fact that a person may occupy many roles points to the desirability of examining combinations as well as individual roles. It is conceivable that certain combinations which involve incompatibilities of striving sentiments may turn out to be particularly significant in creating conditions that foster psychiatric disorder.

In all of the above, societies are regarded as performing their functions well above the level of survival, even if some of them do so more effectively than others. When it was said that one culture might be more efficient than another, it was visualized that both would be operating as effectively as their own standards require, even if one might, for instance, have occasional famine. It is proposed now that attention be given to a society that is performing badly according to its own standards, namely a society that is relatively lacking in integration and consequently failing to carry out its primary functions. Obviously, an extreme condition of this sort cannot last indefinitely; but it can last for a time, and a somewhat less severely hampered but nevertheless defective society may last for a considerable period.

Examples of disintegration are evident in societies that have been disrupted by forced migration, wars, economic disaster, industrial revolution, and extremely rapid acculturation. As a result, defects appear in the patterns of communication, leadership, followership, and cooperation; and failures occur in the functions concerned with the provisions of food, shelter, and clothing, the protection of health, the maintenance of law and order, defense against enemies, the care of children, the satisfaction of emotional needs, and other functions essential to the survival and welfare of the society.

It is evident that marked failure of sociocultural integration in a society will produce severe interference with most of the essential striving sentiments. Thus, physical security, opportunities to give and receive love, the achievement of recognition, the expression of creativity, orientation in regard to one's place in society, membership in a definite human group, and the sense of belonging to a moral order are all apt to be adversely affected, many of them sweepingly so. Similarly, opportunities for the formation and perpetuation of many symptom patterns tend to become wide open, while resources for healthy patterns of adaptation through stable leadership and institutions are generally reduced.

It is evident, also, that in highly disintegrated societies the number of individuals involved will be large. In extreme cases virtually the entire population will be affected, although to varying degrees. If the condition lasts for a number of years, not only are previously normal, fully developed personalities put under stress, but there is every likelihood that, through impingement on infants and children, malformation of developing personalities will result.

The last point pertains to the idea that personality is an integrate unit composed of learned sentiments that are rooted in the emotions, drives, cognitive abilities, and experience of the person and are represented in mentation and in the negotiation of interpersonal relations by symbols. The process of malformation may be outlined as follows: The family as a social institution within the society suffers disintegration. As a consequence, the actions and attitudes of the mother and father deviate markedly from those that are ideal and functional for parents in that society and culture. The parental and other related symbols and sentiments are correspondingly distorted in the developing child, and a personality results which will have great difficulty in later adjustment because of defective organization of sentiments involving men, women, love, authority, and numerous other aspects of life. In short, disintegration of society means disintegration of symbol and sentiment formation; malformed personalities are laid down in malfunctioning societies.

This is another way of saying that social disintegration interferes with the definition of adequate objects and the development of adequate essential striving sentiments. Doubtless much of the effect on the individual can be reversed later by more benign—that is, integrated— social environment, but it seems likely that some defect of personality might remain.

Perhaps the most intriguing aspect of social disintegration as a framework for studying the distribution of psychiatric disorder is the possibility of separating the effects of heredity and the effects of the social environment. If it should be found that there is a high correlation between psychiatric disorder and social disintegration, then it ought to be possible to study a series of groups in which the disintegrating forces come from outside the society and can in no very plausible way be connected with heredity defect of the constituent members. Should it be found that groups of people disintegrated by forced migration or extremely rapid social change or by other such extraneous factors have a higher incidence or prevalence of psychiatric disorder than matched groups from the same culture who have not undergone these experiences, then there would be evidence of environmental effects.

For the above reasons, together with considerations of practicability, the social integration-disintegration approach has been given emphasis in the Stirling County Study.

APPENDIX

The major assumptions on which this frame of reference is based are here brought together in the form of propositions for the purpose of highlighting their interrelationships. Series A states the fundamental proposition regarding the essential psychical condition; Series B and C deal with the nature and direction of response to disturbance of the essential psychical condition; Series D, E, and F concern the manner in which the essential psychical condition may be disturbed; and Series G and H delineate the relationship of social environment to the disturbance of the essential psychical condition and to its consequences.

Series A. The Fundamental Propositions

A1. All human beings exist in a state of psychological striving.
A2. Striving plays a part in the maintenance of an essential psychical condition.
A3. Interference with striving leads to a disturbance of the essential psychical condition.
A4. Disturbance of the essential psychical condition gives rise to disagreeable feelings.

Series B. Propositions Concerned with the Evolution of a Psychiatric Disorder

B1. Given a disturbance of the essential psychical condition, a personality may adopt patterns of sentiment and action which lead to some relief from the resultant disagreeable feelings (A4), but which fail to restore adequately the essential psychical condition.

B2. Because of the relief, each response facilitates its repetition: hence there is a tendency for a personality to persist in a maladaptive direction (B1) once this has been started, leading ultimately to the occurrence of psychiatric disorders.

B3. Given a disturbance of the essential psychical condition (A4), physiological symptoms may appear as part of a general disturbance of dynamic equilibrium in the organism.

B4. Given a disturbance of the essential psychical condition (A4), pre-existing defect in personality may contribute toward the development of psychiatric disorder and/or the appearance of physiological symptoms.

B5. Given a disturbance of the essential psychical condition (A4), sociocultural conditions have a selective influence on the emergence and persistence of malfunctional patterns of personality leading to psychiatric disorder (B1, B2, and B3).

Series C. Propositions Concerned with the Nonoccurrence of Psychiatric Disorder

C1. Given a disturbance of the essential psychical condition a personality may adopt patterns of sentiment and action which lead to relief of the resultant disagreeable feelings (A4), by means of restoration of the essential psychical condition.

C2. Because of the relief, each response facilitates its repetition, hence there is a tendency for a personality system to persist in the constructive direction (C1) once this has been started, leading to adequate, or even superior functioning.

C3. Given a resolution of the disturbance to the essential psychical condition, and a consequent improvement in dynamic equilibrium of the organism, there will be nonoccurrence or disappearance of psychophysiological disorders.

C4. Given a disturbance of the essential psychical condition (A4), pre-existing resources of the personality may contribute toward the development of adequate or superior functioning.

C5. Given a disturbance of the essential psychical condition (A4), sociocultural conditions have a selective influence on the emergence and persistence of personality patterns which do not lead to psychiatric disorder and which may lead to superior functioning (C1, C2, and C3).

Series BC. Combined Proposition

BC1. The trends indicated for the development of psychiatric disorder (B1, B2, B3, and B4) and for the maintenance of health or increasing capabilities (C1, C2, C3, and C4) can occur simultaneously in the same personality.

Series D. Propositions Concerning Interference with the Essential Striving Sentiments

D1. Given Proposition A2 certain striving sentiments may be designated as essential because maximally concerned with the maintenance of the "essential" psychical condition.

D2. Essential striving sentiments may fail in this function due to interference imposed by the environment.

D3. Essential striving sentiments may fail in this function due to defects inherent in the objects of striving.

D4. Essential striving sentiments may fail in this function due to defect, inborn or acquired, in the personality.

Series E. Propositions Relating Essential Striving
Sentiments and Sociocultural Environment

E1. Sociocultural situations which interfere with sentiments of physical security foster psychiatric disorder.

E2. Sociocultural situations which interfere with sentiments of securing sexual satisfaction foster psychiatric disorder.

E3. Sociocultural situations which interfere with sentiments bearing on the expression of hostility foster psychiatric disorder.

E4. Sociocultural situations which interfere with sentiments of giving love foster psychiatric disorder.

E5. Sociocultural situations which interfere with sentiments of securing love foster psychiatric disorder.

E6. Sociocultural situations which interfere with sentiments bearing on obtaining recognition foster psychiatric disorder.

E7. Sociocultural situations which interfere with sentiments bearing on the expression of spontaneity (positive force, creativity, volition) foster psychiatric disorder.

E8. Sociocultural situations which interfere with sentiments of orientation in the person regarding his place in society and the place of others foster psychiatric disorder.

E9. Sociocultural situations which interfere with the person's sentiments of membership in a definite human group foster psychiatric disorder.

E10. Sociocultural situations which interfere with sentiments of belonging to a moral order and of being right in what one does foster psychiatric disorder.

Series F. Proposition Relating Interpersonal Patterns
and Sociocultural Environment

F1. Sociocultural situations which expose a growing personality to defective role relationships foster psychiatric disorder.

Series G. Propositions Regarding the Nature of
Society and Culture

G1. Human society is composed of a network of interrelated sociocultural self-integrating units.

G2. Each self-integrating unit is an energy system and is in a constant state of performing functions upon which its existence depends.

G3. The functioning of the unit as a unit (G2) proceeds through patterns of interpersonal relationships based on the communication of shared symbols and coordinating sentiments.

Series H. Propositions Relating Sociocultural Patterns
to Psychiatric Disorder

H1. Given that human society is composed of functioning self-integrating units based on patterns of interpersonal relationships which include communications, symbols, and sentiments (G series), it follows that the different functional parts of a particular unit (such as associations, socio-economic classes, and roles) may have differential effects on personalities exposed to them and hence on mental health (B5, C5, D3, E series, and F).

H2. Given that human society is composed of functioning self-integrating units based on patterns of interpersonal relationships which include communication, symbols, and sentiments (G series), it follows that different units with different patterns of organization (culture) may have differential effects on personalities exposed to them and hence on mental health (B5, C5, D2, D3, E series, and F).

H3. Given that human society is composed of functioning self-integrating units based on patterns of interpersonal relationships which include communications, symbols, and sentiments (G series), it follows that social disintegration will affect personalities in such a manner as to foster psychiatric disorder (B5, C5, D2, D3, E series, and F).

This paper was adapted by the author from Psychiatric disorder and social environment, *Psychiatry, 18* (No. 4) Nov. 1955, and *My name is legion,* Foundations for a Theory of Man in Relation to Culture (Volume I, The Stirling County Study of Psychiatric Disorder and Sociocultural Environment). New York: Basic Books, 1959. Reprinted by special permission of the William Alanson White Psychiatric Foundations, Inc., and Basic Books, Inc., Copyrights William Alanson White Foundations, Inc., 1955, and Basic Books, Inc., 1959.

5

The Empirical Status of the Integration-Disintegration Hypothesis

DOROTHEA C. LEIGHTON, M.D.

The preceding chapter has stated at length the various dimensions of the integration-disintegration hypothesis, its effect upon the essential striving sentiments, and its relationship to the development of psychiatric disorder. The Stirling County study [1] was the first proving ground of this hypothesis and furnished evidence that, in a population subdivided for the most part into small quasi-organismic communities, the quality of the socio-cultural environment, whether integrated or the reverse, appeared to be strongly associated with better or poorer mental health, respectively. There was an English and a French integrated community and three small ethnically mixed disintegrated communities, which provided strong contrast in the proportion of the population that showed evidence of psychiatric disorder and of mental health. If, for example, the mean value for the County as a whole (both sexes) is .50, the chance that an individual member of a subgroup will show psychiatric disorder is as follows:

	Disintegrated communities	English integrated	French integrated	Whole county
Men	.68	.43	.47	.44
Women	.65	.60	.40	.55

Whole county probability = .50

[1] This study is reported chiefly in the following three volumes: Leighton, Alexander H. *My name is legion.* New York: Basic Books, 1959; Hughes, Charles

In addition, an extension of the Stirling County study to 15 villages in Nigeria provided a further opportunity to test the hypothesis [2]. Although it is not easy to characterize communities in a little known culture on the integration dimension, the counsel of numerous Nigerian advisors and assistants made it feasible to attempt such a distinction, with results very similar to the Stirling County findings. That is, there was a considerably heightened proportion of psychiatric disorder in the villages judged (in advance) to be disintegrated, and a larger proportion of mental health in the integrated villages.

Let us examine, then, how the various indicators of integration-disintegration, as seen in these two studies, actually were related to the increase of psychiatric disorder or the preservation of mental health. First in order is physical security, which can be stated as:

> Hypothesis 1: Socio-cultural disintegration fosters psychiatric disorder by interfering with physical security—e.g., needs for adequate food, shelter, clothing, sleep, and care of physical ailments.

This aspect of sociocultural disintegration is commonly associated with poverty, which was certainly a striking characteristic of the disintegrated communities in Stirling County. In Nigeria the difference between villages was less outstanding, but even so, there were more tumbledown houses, more trash lying around, and less evidence that the inhabitants had been able to afford such imported luxuries as an alarm clock in the disintegrated villages.

Additional evidence from military psychiatry reinforces the notion that lack of physical supports undermines the ability of soldiers to endure the hazards of warfare, especially if it persists for a long period of time [3]. It is said to lead to ineffectiveness as a soldier under

C. et al. People of cove and woodlot. New York: Basic Books, 1960; Leighton, Dorothea C. et al. The character of danger. New York: Basic Books, 1963.

[2] Leighton, A. H., Lambo, T. A., Hughes, C. C., Leighton, D. C., Murphy, J. M., & Macklin, D. B. Psychiatric disorder among the Yoruba. Ithaca: Cornell University Press, 1963.

[3] Ginsburg, E., Anderson, J. K., Ginsburg, S. W., Herma, J. L., Bray, D. W., Jordan, W., & Ryan, F. J. Patterns of performance. Vol. III, The ineffective soldier. New York: Columbia University Press, 1959, P. 42.

combat conditions, and it seems to contribute to ineffectiveness as a citizen elsewhere.

An unexpected finding in Stirling County was that the few individuals living in disintegrated communities who had adequate economic resources (storekeepers, etc.) tended to share the poorer mental health of their neighbors rather than the better mental health of their economic peers. Thus it appears that it is not poverty alone that is the etiologic agent, but a complex of factors of which poverty is one. This is in keeping with occasional observations of excellent morale persisting in the face of temporary economic disaster such as the depression years of 1929 onward.

It can be said categorically that, in general, there is a close relationship between adequacy of physical resources and better mental health, yet the exceptions noted indicate that the matter is considerably more complex than such a statement seems to imply.

> Hypothesis 2: Socio-cultural disintegration fosters mental health by the degree to which it permits freedom of sexual expression.

Freud and the advertising industry have succeeded in convincing many people that this hypothesis is essentially axiomatic. In Stirling County, however, there is much more sexual restraint in the integrated than the disintegrated communities, while in Nigeria sexual restraint is comparatively rare in any community. It appears, then, that physical sex does not greatly promote mental health. It may well be that residents of disintegrated communities would be even worse off if sexual restraints were added to their other shortages. However, it seems more likely that we have taken for the whole picture what is in truth a relatively small part of it—and that the "whole picture" in this case includes much of the supportive network of social and familial interrelationships that, to be sure, regulate the freedom of sexual expression but that may not necessarily be adequately present when sexual expression is unrestrained.

In short, this hypothesis appeared to be unsupported in the two studies cited.

> Hypothesis 3: Socio-cultural disintegration fosters mental health by the degree to which it permits freedom of hostile and aggressive expression.

Freedom of expression of hostile and aggressive feelings is not well tolerated by human groups—or perhaps by groups of other animals either. It is felt as a threat to group cohesiveness and interferes with group consensus and action. It is certainly rife in the disintegrated communities that were studied while it was quite low-keyed and well controlled, although present, in integrated communities. There were few interferences with its expression beyond the danger of reprisal in disintegrated groups, yet this did not seem to offer any substantial protection against psychiatric disorder. It seemed, in fact, to be further divisive of an already divided group.

Thus it appears that neither freedom of sexual expression nor freedom of expression of hostile and aggressive feelings function to promote mental health. Rather, the implication of extensive individual freedom and lack of regulation in itself constitutes an interference with achieving stable socio-cultural patterns for the group and thus interferes with other essential striving sentiments.

> Hypothesis 4: Socio-cultural disintegration fosters psychiatric disorder due to limitations put on the giving and receiving of love.

The absence of warm interpersonal feelings, which is another way of saying the absence of love, is a common accompaniment of the broken homes, few associations, overt hostility, and poor communication by means of which we characterize socio-cultural disintegration. The presence of such feelings, by contrast, inclines individuals to take an interest in each other and to promote each other's well-being.

The difference between integrated and disintegrated communities in respect to this hypothesis is very striking in Stirling County. We were not able to assess it adequately in the Nigerian villages, but its common association with the indicators mentioned above, which we were better able to detect, leads us to conclude that love was present where socio-cultural integration was apparent.

The place where the effect of love showed most clearly was in intrafamilial relationships and attitudes. Families in disintegrated communities were "irregular" in their composition by North American standards. If both husband and wife were present, the children were likely to be either his or hers but not theirs, and sexual relations were likely to be frequently extramarital. Inconsistency of emotional tone was also common, with more tendency toward hostility or neutrality than toward warmth and support. The opposite emotional climate prevailed in integrated communities—"regular" families, joint children, cordial relations between members, expression of predominantly positive rather than negative feelings toward each other.

Thus, more than any factor discussed in the preceding hypotheses, the presence or absence of love seems to be consistently associated with socio-cultural integration or disintegration, respectively. Interference with love appears as a feature that distinguishes between noxious and benign human environments. In many respects this is the obverse of freedom of expression of aggressive or hostile feelings, and it seems to be more powerful in its effect on personality functioning than either sexual satisfaction or physical security.

> Hypothesis 5: Social disintegration fosters psychiatric disorder by interfering with the achievement of socially valued ends by legitimate means.

This is another way of stating the need for recognition, and the interference is associated with poverty, inadequate development of leadership, lack of associations, and poor communications. "Socially valued ends" are not readily available to people in lower socio-economic levels, at least in Western society, even though people at all levels tend to desire power, prestige, and possessions. "Legitimate means" in middle class terms include hard work, frugality, sobriety, politeness, honesty, energy, and intelligence. Application of these means is expected to result in the valued ends, and this provides recognition automatically. The syndrome, of which poverty is a part, provides a very poor base for the operation of the means to attain the end.

Merton [4] distinguishes four main types of individual response to this combination of social ideal and means of achievement. The first of these is *Conformity*, in which the individual works away at trying to achieve the ideal and is rewarded by a certain amount of recognition for modest results, even if in addition he develops a fair number of psychiatric symptoms.

A second type of response is *Innovation-Rebellion*, in which the goals are maintained but the means used are not socially approved— exemplified by a professional criminal or a dishonest business man. When rebellion predominates, there is usually a redefinition of the goals and means such as happens in a delinquent subculture. Attainment of prestige, power, and possessions are still the final goal but may result from activity considered socio-pathic by the middle class and may consist in quite different components when achieved.

A third response is *Ritualism*, whereby the individual slogs away at the means but never expects to achieve the goals. The wage slave, sharecropper, domestic worker, or household drudge are examples of such types, who may often develop mild depression or anxiety.

The final, fourth, reaction is *Retreatism*, which means that the individual (realistically) gives up either following the means or envisioning the goals. The resultant effort to escape problems often enough ends up as alcoholism.

Merton believes that poverty reduces the likelihood of Conformity as a response and increases the likelihood of all the others; this tends to

[4] Merton, Robert *Social theory and social structure*. 2nd ed.; Glencoe: The Free Press, 1957, Chap. IV.

cut individuals off from the mainstream of society. Conformity, as an effort to identify with society's norms, benefits its adherents by providing a sense of belonging both to the group and to a moral order that justifies the required efforts, while the other three types of response set individuals apart from the majority. Thus Conformity tends to protect *from* psychiatric disorder, while the rest conduce toward it.

In the integrated communities, Conformity is the modal response, while in the disintegrated it is very rare. Innovation-Rebellion are common in depressed areas if one accepts as evidence such behavior as amateur theft, poaching, and occasional bootlegging. It may well be, however, that they represent more the gratification of impulses than anything as "conscious" as Innovation-Rebellion. Ritualism is very rare in disintegrated communities while Retreatism is very common.

Thus Hypothesis 5 offers a plausible process whereby poverty affecting a whole community might be expected to influence the prevalence of psychiatric disorder by altering the possible life styles of the residents. There are few examples of "approved" modes of response and many of the nonapproved. Assuming that young people tend to pattern themselves on the models provided by their elders, it is to be expected that in disintegrated communities the nonsupportive responses prevail while in the integrated communities it is more "natural" to conform to the response approved by the larger society. One wonders what might result if the disintegrated group should come to feel that its patterns of response were proper and worthwhile.

Hypothesis 6: Socio-cultural disintegration fosters psychiatric disorder by interfering with spontaneity.

"Spontaneity," "positive force," "creativity," or "volition" are thought of as variously representing the concept here. It seems curious that lack of social restraints, which are commonly believed to cramp the qualities listed, should not result in a burgeoning of creativity. Such is by no means the case, however, although there are individual exceptions. Along with material poverty, secularization, lack of leadership, and lack of associations to belong to, there seems to be a poverty of enthusiasm that produces an atmosphere of apathy. Even the things that people "like to do" seem to be in default of anything better—sex, aggression, drinking, and doing nothing.

The disintegrated communities provide few opportunities, few models, and few rewards for creativity or meaningful choices. The person who feels a creative urge must steel himself against the almost inevitable ridicule, somehow mustering individual courage to do what he wants. The rare "healthy" person has discovered how to get enjoyment out of what he does. By contrast, the cultural climate of the integrated communities appears more tolerant and rewarding of originality, and more encouraging of the expression of feelings and ideas, which seems to serve to protect and promote mental health of its inhabitants. Altogether, various aspects of disintegration appear to damp down spontaneity and thus to require a much greater "head of steam" to permit any substantial creative expression.

> Hypothesis 7: Social disintegration fosters psychiatric disorder by interfering with a person's orientation regarding his place in society;
>
> Hypothesis 8: and with his sense of membership in a definite human group.

These two interrelated hypotheses go with few and weak associations, lack of leadership, and inadequate communication. One might well say that Hypothesis 7 does not apply, for residents of disintegrated communities have quite a clear impression that their place is at the very bottom of society. The only people lower than a given member of such a community are the other members, and each person feels himself rather alone. The striking lack of voluntary associations (as compared with the integrated communities) and the high level of hostility and of minor crime and delinquency give little for a person to identify with. One might conclude that the difficulty residents of disintegrated communities experience in "sticking it out" in unfamiliar other kinds of communities indicates that they have strongly identified with their place of origin. Evidence favors more the probability that they cannot stand the other community because of lack of techniques for association rather than from loyalty to the community of origin: They feel more comfortable where everybody behaves as they do.

Three of the leading sentiments of the disintegrated areas—"people here are mentally and morally inferior"; "people are changeable and shifty, and you have to stand by yourself in life"; and "it is good to be with people but you have to watch your step"—give the key suggestion that it is not so much lack of orientation as it is that the consequences of their orientation are very different from that of people in integrated communities, due in large part, it seems, to interferences with both the striving sentiments toward love and toward recognition. While there is considerable doubt that the group to which disintegrated community members belong is a very definite one, still it is less lack of belonging than lack of satisfaction in belonging that is the crux of the matter. It is a combination of alienation and disparagement which leads to some feeling of isolation even at home, and to much greater aloneness everywhere else.

Hypothesis 9: Social disintegration fosters psychiatric disorder by interfering with the individual's sense of membership in a moral order.

This hypothesis is related to the indicator definitions: cultural confusion, secularization, lack of membership in associations, lack of leaders, and inadequate communications. The moral order that the member of a disintegrated community dimly perceives is a watered-down version of the values of the dominant society, which, his experience tells him, do not work in his setting. The principal contribution of this is to intensify the feeling of inferiority vis-a-vis residents of nondisintegrated parts of the county.

On the sociological side, however, there is a pronounced effect that has been discussed by Durkheim and interpreted by Talbott Parsons as follows:

> Not merely contractual relations but stable social relations
> in general and even the personal equilibrium of the
> members of a social group are seen to be dependent on the
> existence of a normative structure in relation to conduct,
> generally accepted as having moral authority by the
> members of the community, and upon their effective
> subordination to these norms. They not merely regulate the
> individual's choice of means to his ends, but his very needs
> and desires themselves are determined in part by them.
> When this controlling normative structure is upset and
> disorganized, individual conduct is equally disorganized and
> chaotic—the individual loses himself in a void of meaning-
> less activities. *Anomie* is precisely this state of disorganiza-
> tion where the hold of norms over individual conduct has
> broken down [5].

Certainly one of the striking differences between the integrated and
disintegrated communities in Stirling County is the presence of
normative values and behavior in the former and their absence in the
latter (as in urban slums). The moral order is mediated strongly by the
religious institutions in the integrated communities and to some extent
also by the economic institutions and the family and kinship systems,
all of which (both institutions and systems) are rather conspicuously
lacking in disintegrated communities. The first two indicator definitions
above, cultural confusion and secularization, refer primarily to anomie
in Durkheim's sense of the term. In justice to Durkheim, however, it
must be noted that he never worked with such a small unit of
population as we have been doing, building his theories for the most
part about whole countries or regions. Furthermore, he felt that
material poverty served as an almost certain guarantee against anomie.
This may have been a more appropriate conclusion in his day than
currently.

In conclusion to this brief condensation of the considerably more
adequate treatment found in Chapter XIII of *The character of danger*,
let us summarize the main points. We can say in the first place that the
various hypotheses proposed in the frame of reference were borne out

[5] Parsons, Talcott, *The structure of social action*. 2nd ed.; Glencoe: The Free
Press, 1949, P. 377.

in varying degrees by the testing of the research. On the whole, the most clearly and directly noxious aspects of socio-cultural disintegration appear to be those that affect the achievement of love, recognition, spontaneity, and the sense of belonging to a moral order and being right in what one does. The importance of the ten indicator-definitions depends on the finding that, alone or in combination, they interfere with such achievements. Somewhat unexpectedly, physical insecurity and the frustration of sexual or aggressive impulses did not appear very important among noxious influences associated with disintegration of the kind investigated.

Finally, since psychiatric disorder is considerably more prevalent and more impairing in disintegrated communities, what aspects of the disintegration foster the emergence of psychiatric disorder from the disturbed essential psychical condition? It seems clear that the noxious influences begin early for the child in the disintegrated situation and recur throughout his life-arc. Needs for security, love, and approval are met only partially and inconsistently, leading to malformation of his personality and to later malfunctioning.

Choices are so limited that substitutions for unobtainable objects are not possible, in addition to which there is little guidance for making the choices so as to avoid unworkable and self-defeating results. Even though the resources of integrated communities are not infallible, they include the helps of tradition, religion, books, magazines, and compassionate advice in great profusion as compared to the disintegrated communities. Thus there is not much to prevent, and there may even be much to encourage a person with a disturbed psychical condition to seek relief by withdrawing into daydreams; building satisfactions on paranoid systems of thought; forgetting the past and blotting out the future; sinking into a chronic state of apathy, depression, and anxiety; or masking the disturbed feelings by the use of alcohol, sex, fighting, stealing, and other forms of excitement.

6

Seminar Assessment of the Integration-Disintegration Framework

.

BERTON H. KAPLAN, Ph.D.

Contributors

Isidor Chein, Ph.D.	Lawrence Hinkle, M.D.
Catherine Fales, M.D.	Laurel Hodgden, Ph.D
William Foote Whyte, Ph.D	Raymond Illsley, Ph.D
John R. P. French, Ph.D	Thomas Langner, Ph.D
Nicholas Freydberg, Ph.D	Alexander H. Leighton, M.D.
John C. Harding, Ph.D	Jane Murphy, Ph.D

The basic purpose of the seminar series was to advance our systematic thinking about the social processes that influence mental health. The first session opened on this comment by Alexander H. Leighton:

> I think the fixed limits of this group are only that we are concerned with social processes relevant to mental health, or relevant to psychiatric disorders. I do not think beyond that we are terribly fixed. Now unfixed, but influential, is our experience and thinking which to date have been in terms of these two concepts: socio-economic status and

social integration-disintegration. We want to re-examine all
of this as freely and frankly as we can, and see if there are
not better ways of putting calipers on nature, or if we are
going to put calipers on nature in these ways, then let's be
more clear about it.

The seminar sessions were thus launched with this invitation to
examine critically the social processes relevant to psychiatric disorder.
Two areas were of paramount importance: (1) a discussion of the social
process that has been labeled integration-disintegration in the Stirling
research (this chapter); and, (2) the social system units that are most
appropriate as units of observation in urban settings (see Chapters
7-11).

The largest part of the following commentary was devoted to a
discussion of the concept of social integration-disintegration. A series of
important questions dominated this discussion: What is social disintegration [1]? When is a person in a disintegrative situation? How do you
account for different individual capacities in a disorganized situation?
How do you distinguish different levels of disintegration—personal,
social, and biological? What are the properties of a noxious or healthy
social situation?

Now, we briefly define and illustrate each of these discussed aspects
of integration-disintegration. In keeping with a working paper type
format, it is assumed that the problems of exhaustiveness of definition
and dimension will not be solved here. However, it is hoped that critical
reactions will generate greater conceptual clarity and fresh hypotheses
about the relationship of the process of integration-disintegration to
mental health.

In responding to the goal of re-examining the independent variable of
integration-disintegration, the following dimensions were extracted
from the seminar discussions:

1. Instrumental disorganization
2. Normative interference

[1] The terms "disintegration" and "disorganization" are both used in the
discussion to follow.

3. Environmental malfunctioning
4. Powerlessness
5. Cueing disturbances
6. Group conflicts
7. Level of integration
8. Need interference
9. Customary pattern interference
10. Resource deprivation
11. Integration and numbers of interaction
12. Social discontinuities
13. Ineffective role-personality allocation

We must emphasize that these categories may overlap. But for the sake of emphasis and the natural history of ideas, we have chosen to preserve the commentaries as they occurred. We also recognize that these dimensions vary as to a focus on the individual or on the system as a whole.

1. INSTRUMENTAL DISORGANIZATION

The seminar discussion demonstrated that there are numerous shades of meaning attached to the concept of integration-disintegration. Chein points out that Merton's views on the concept of anomie could be labeled as "essential instrumental disorganization," that is, people have goals but no ways of satisfying them. Chein (Seminar 1, p. 12) stated:

Merton plays up an obvious one in his version of the concept of anomie as the essential instrumental disorganization. People have goals. If there is no way of satisfying them, that is one form of disintegration. It is not necessarily having people getting in your way or having conflicting directions.

2. NORMATIVE INTERFERENCE

Chein also referred to normative interference as a type of disintegration. What does an individual want in his particular context? What does he see himself doing? What gets in his way? What kinds of demands are being made upon him? What is he ready or unready to accept?

Chein (Seminar 1, p. 14) points out that normative disintegration involves the following:

It seems to me that the disorganization issue, once you focus on an individual, always comes down to the use of his time. What gets in his way? What's pushing him around?

Furthermore, as Chein points out, you can focus on the individual's view of social disintegration by studying commitments, barriers to goal attainment, and the degree to which the normative structure issues conflicting directions (Seminar 1, pp. 38-40).

(*Social process*: Can focus on individual's view of social disintegration by determining the extent that barriers get in way of what he's committed to doing and degree of normative structure issuing conflicting direction.)

Chein: It seems to me that the nature of the questions of "why" goes to the heart of the issue of the relation of mental illness to society.

I would say that the guy who is in solitary confinement will become sick if he finds nothing to sustain any of the activities to which he is committed. If, in this situation, he can pursue these activities, then he's in isolation. I think this is just as true if he's in solitary as if he's in the community but not of it. If he's in a work situation but can carry on whatever it is that he wants to carry on in work situations, there's nothing disruptive in isolation *per se*. It's disruptive if, in some way, there's something that gets in the way of doing the things that he's committed to doing, which helps to focus the issue of what social disorganization is. At least from this perspective, if one starts from the individual, there are other people who get in his way, and he can't carry things through because there are constantly barriers interposed by the things that other people are doing. In one sense, you have social disorganization where everybody gets in everybody's way. You have an army. The army is supposed to move from here to there. But every time you start out in one direction somebody else is in your way, so you start out in some other direction, and pretty soon you don't know where you're going.

What's more, if you start out to go with somebody in particular, i.e., your goal is not just to get there by yourself, but along with somebody else, pretty soon you find yourself separated from that somebody else. It's simply a function of people's getting into each other's way. There, the supportive system that makes the behavior possible vanishes, and in such a situation a person becomes lost if it is possible for other people to get in his way. Right there is where one gets into the other aspect of the integration issue; namely, the normative structure, the demands that are made on the individual to act thus and so. You have a total state of social disorganization when the normative structure is pulling the individual in conflicting directions and nobody may be getting in his way. To take an old illustration of Karen Horney's: if I have committed myself in terms of a normative structure to brotherly love, and if I also have committed myself to beating everybody, I am in trouble, and I have to resolve this in some way. There have to be normative outlets which will keep individuals from getting into trouble, but the directions are directions that say: "go in these opposite or mutually conflicting ways."

From here on, granted that this individual does spend this proportion of his time in such a context and that portion of his time in another kind of context, it becomes essentially a question of what are the properties of these various contexts in which he spends his time and in which presumably spending time means he is doing something. Are other people getting in his way and is he being given conflicting directions?

Normative interferences can also be studied in terms of *internalized* conflicts.

Chein: It is proscriptions that get in my way. They not only get in my way, but when I internalize these, they're no longer coming from society; I have them already, and at this point now, I find that these proscriptions get in the way of my fulfilling these internalized commitments. I am never just hungry. At the same time that I am hungry or can anticipate hunger, I am also somebody who needs recognition; I am also somebody who needs security; I am also somebody who needs status; I am also somebody who needs a sure position so I know where I am; I'm also somebody who has to be helpful to people, and I keep getting into trouble because I want to be helpful.

3. ENVIRONMENTAL MALFUNCTIONING

In examining the problem of integration-disintegration, it is possible to focus on the whole system. In this case, we assume that the environment that is not functioning properly is potentially pathogenic. The following observations on this view of integration-disintegration were made (Seminar 1, pp. 2-5):

(*Focus on individual*: Environment not properly functioning is potentially pathogenic.)

Chein: I think I looked at it (disintegration) from a different angle. With regard to the question of mental illness, I asked what kind of environment is pathogenic? An environment that isn't properly functioning is potentially pathogenic, and this would be just as true of group functioning. We wouldn't ordinarily think of these as sick, but it's essentially the same issue, the issue of properly functioning. I take as a premise that functional interference in matters with which one is concerned is a prime requisite for a pathogenic environment. If there's an out, this isn't pathogenic, but if you're confronted with an existence in which you can anticipate the recurrence of a crisis without being able to anticipate the possibility of being able to cope with this recurring crisis, this kind of thing would be disruptive, or at least impose a challenge and call for more than usual resources on the part of the human being in order to cope with such a situation.

(*Focus on social unit*: Anything in way of *group's* long-term commitments is disruptive.)

The same thing would apply to groups insofar as groups have long-range commitments. Anything that gets in the way of these long-range commitments, activities, programs, and what not is going to be disruptive to the organization or to the group, and so one gets at the level of organization. Perhaps what I call a social disintegration is a situation when what is approved in one group interferes with the organization within another group. When one takes a social context that interferes with the individual's organization, at another level, this is what I think would be a property of a pathogenic environment.

(*Focus on individual*: Kind of things that get in way: people interfering, lack of means, difficulty in communication.)

Then, I say to myself: What kind of things can get in the way of the functioning of an individual? Literally, people get in his way because when he tries to do something there is always somebody interfering. Another thing would be when the means of carrying out his long-range programs don't exist or are difficult to use and in that way interfere with the individual's functioning, as, for example, what I'd refer to as a "cue system." In order to be able to carry out my activities, insofar as I'm dependent upon others, I've got to be able to communicate with them; anything that would interfere with communication would interfere with the activities. If we bring a bunch of people together from a variety of disciplines, and they are unable to communicate, the whole system would go haywire.

This isn't pathogenic because it is circumscribed. If they have to function together for a long enough period of time, they'll acquire the capacity to be communicative. But there are other kinds of things that get in the way of the adjustment of the "cueing system" and that have long-range effects.

(*Focus on individual*: Interdependence of various commitments and disruptive effect of change in this pattern.)

I start with an assumption that the various commitments of an individual are themselves interdependent with other things, so my seeking of security is not independent of what my relationship is to my competency, or what my relationship is to the seeking of recognition. These fit into each other.

Then encountering an environmental situation in which the pattern of interdependencies change—the ways in which I achieve security are no longer compatible with the way in which I receive integration, this now requires a complete reintegration on my part. Insofar as this involves a long-range integration, I become incapable of functioning until I am capable of achieving the new integration, which in my terms would be achieving a new personality.

(Focus: The question is: What are properties of environmental illness?)

Chein (from Seminar 1, pp. 27-28): It seems to me that the focus of the study is quite clear. You have an individual who develops hallucinations, delusions, anxieties, depressions, compulsions, or what have you, and the nature of the question is: Given that there are many such individuals, what are the properties of the environment in which they move that contribute to the generation of these conditions? From this point of view, it seems to me the focus is always clear. *It is not the question: Are his personal, his interpersonal relationships disorganized? It is the question: Does he move in an environment that is disorganized from a social point of view?* It is not asking whether there may be other kinds of contributors to the development of these conditions. The poisoned atmosphere that we live in may or may not make a difference with regard to the functioning of individuals or their likelihood of developing, if they're in some other kind of trouble, if they're in some other kind of trouble, hallucinations, depressions, etc.

The focus of the question is that people move in a social environment. The working hypothesis is that when they encounter disorganization, they get into trouble; this trouble is something that helps to account for etiology of their mental illness, and that seems to me to be the focus.

4. POWERLESSNESS

In considering another dimension of disintegration, the question was raised whether a central factor in the transaction between the individual and his environment is the person's perception of his power or powerlessness. Freydberg (Seminar 1, p. 15) offered the following hypothesis:

(*Social process*: Possible central factor, person's perception of own power.)

Freydberg: I wonder if there is a kind of central factor in these aspects, a person's perception of his own power or powerlessness, and the degree to which this seems to be affected by someone getting in his way, or some value system that he cannot meet, such as goals of the society that are unattainable. His mental health seems to be related to the extent that he is rendered powerless by such events.

5. CUEING DISTURBANCES

Another way in which integration-disintegration may be observed is in face-to-face relationships. In fact, the "cueing system" is one way in which to study aspects of integration or disintegration.

Chein refers to two dimensions of cueing disturbance: clarity of expectations and communicative clarity (the Tower of Babel problem).

(*Focus*: Question is, when is person in disintegrating situation?)

Chein: Well, if you start with your focus on the individual, the question is when is a person in a disintegrated situation? The disintegration may manifest itself in his face-to-face relationships. Take the cueing system. Perhaps he cannot tell from the other individuals when to do things that will fit in with what they are doing in their face-to-face interactions, or perhaps he doesn't know whether he is in a situation vis-a-vis the other individual in which, to take a normative example, he is supposed to act in act in a symmetrical manner or in a complementary manner. What is expected of him?

Face-to-face relationships do not necessarily take the form of any kind of formally distinguished group structures, but if he is dealing with people who do not know how to communicate their needs, he is in trouble wherever he confronts such individuals. Take a psychiatrist who is faced by a patient. This is a disintegrated dyad if he can't tell what his patient is saying to him, whether it is expression, behavior, or language. If he gets the key to this, if the cueing system starts functioning, it does not matter whether he pursues a formal language, he knows what the other guy means. Take the classical example of disintegration, the Tower of Babel. Nobody knew what anybody else was saying, and they were all in trouble, but they were in trouble in terms of interpersonal relations.

You have individuals interacting with groups as groups, where it does not matter who the other individuals are. I have responsibilities to my class, and these responsibilities remain constant regardless of who happens to be in the class. I find myself, in a system in which my function is supposed to be to review whatever text materials they use because eventually my class is going to get the same examination that other people's classes are going to get. I also discover that my function is supposed to be to bring out their creativeness; in this situation, I am in trouble because I have conflicting demands on me, and they are not vis-a-vis individuals. They are vis-a-vis an abstract bunch of people, a group.

I can also find myself in some relationship to different kinds of institutions. I guess one could make a systematic classification of this sort of thing and define what the nature of institutional disorganizations would be. What are the things that disrupt my interactions as a person versus other persons, other groups, institutions, etc.?

Now, if you were to go about measuring this organization per se rather than taking indirect indices, I suppose one could take a sample of people in special departments, areas, etc., throughout the building, and gather them all up and you have an index.

6. GROUP CONFLICTS

In studying disintegration, if the focus is on the group, you can look at the conflicting demands between groups. Group members can be asked to do things that are not consistent. For example, we can find an individual who acts for the group caught between demands that are obviously inconsistent. In fact, his actions can get the group into trouble no matter how well integrated the group is internally. Chein (Seminar 1, pp. 18-19) observed:

(*Focus*: Same can be said for groups as for individuals.)

Chein: I could show the exact same thing focusing on groups because they are in situations vis-a-vis one another in which they have conflicting demands, conflicting needs, and they get in the way of each other. Take the police and the social workers. I can sympathize with Police Commissioner Murphy who once declared that all these social workers were trying to make social workers out of the police. Now he is not representative of a group that has an assigned social function, that has been defined in a particular way but it is constantly being redefined by the demands that other segments of society are making on the police. He finds that his group is being asked to do things that are not mutually consistent; if he agrees, the group is in trouble. It is a disorganized setup, whatever its internal structure is, which may or may not be organized.

However you define a community, I think the larger the units that you get into, the fewer the areas of possible disorganization develop. You can take a nation, it is in a disorganized world if it never knows what it can count upon from other nations. If it is in a setup in which the expectations and the demands of all nations are clearly defined, you know what to expect, you have a good communications system, you have good means of pursuing your ends while they pursue their ends without getting in each other's way, then it's Utopia. It is a well-organized world, and at that level again, it seems to me, talking about nations, the issue is one in which you know the possibility of organizaton or disorganization.

In any event, community is not the right word, rather a legally defined subgroup. You have the schools, the police, and the churches. If people find themselves in situations in which schools are pushing them in one direction, the community agencies are pushing them in another direction, and the churches are saying to them, "things in this world don't matter, think about the other world," and everybody is pulling in opposite directions on an institutional level, the individual may be in a bad spot because that kind of disorganization will reflect itself in terms of his individual situation.

7. LEVEL OF INTEGRATION

In the seminar discussion, it was also pointed out that it is very important to distinguish *levels* of integration-disintegration in terms of individuals, institutions, and society. For example, you can have a situation in which the husband meets his goals in a way that denies the wife her goals. You can also have situations in which something may be integrative for institutions but not for the individuals within it. What is integrative for society is not the same as asking what is integrative for the individual. The point is: it is important to distinguish levels of integration. Illsley's (Seminar 2, p. 26) and Hinkle's (Seminar 2, p. 27) comments are very relevant.

(*Focus*: Important to distinguish integrative for institution and for individual.)

Illsley: Let's take an example here. Let's take a problem that's likely to flare up fairly acutely in a society such as Manhattan where you've got a large number of people coming into the society, the out-of-towners—shall we say the professional groups—coming into the society and seeking jobs. For them, one of their goals is success in their careers. This may be shared between the husband and the wife. It may be necessary, too, from the point of view of an institution, the work institution, that people should move around in this way, to get the right kind of person in the right kind of place at the right kind of time. He comes into Manhattan, and he may get a great deal of satisfaction out of the work he does.

However, he brings his dependents into this situation where they themselves may find, particularly if this is a recurrent process, moving around from one group to another, from one area to another, disintegration of the family relationships, and of the relationships of these people to people in society at large. You may have here two institutions, the family and work, which are each in a way attempting to integrate themselves, but which are mutually contradictory.

I can see where it becomes important to distinguish between what is integration for an institution, or for a system, and what is integrative for the individual.

(*Focus*: Asking what's integrative for society not same as what's for individual.)

Hinkle: I go along with this very much. I think what you are saying is that you may have a large community and a large social system that is perhaps integrating and growing, and in the process of integrating, it may be disintegrating to certain aspects of the individuals' lives. However, what you study depends on your viewpoint when you ask the question. I would not necessarily assume that the phenomena of integration or disintegration in a society, or in a subsection, is the same thing as disintegration of interpersonal relations.

8. PERSONALITY NEED INTERFERENCE

In the continuing discussion of the concepts of integration-disintegration, Fales asked this question: How are individual needs satisfied in the community or group? For this point of view the problem is to focus on needs. The focus is on the question of whether people are living in communities and subgroups that satisfy personality needs, for example, affiliative needs. As Langner points out: What would a community be like if it were in line with the individual's needs? Fales (Seminar 2, p. 31) and Langner (Seminar 2, p. 31-32) observed:

Fales: Do you think it is actually possible to define a series of communities in a city as large as New York, or an area or a group of people as complex and varied as this? I was struck by a group of telephone operators; each of them went back to very parallel types of relationships or equivalent relationships. Could one set up some such set that a person needs, to have so many particularly integrated, or tightly organized, or well organized types of relationships? I am thinking in terms of the individual and working from there. I am so struck with the thought of the great deal of emphasis here on drive, and less on needs. I wonder very much if this question of integrated people belonging to a great many organizations in an integrated community does not satisfy many affiliated needs. Possibly you could go back to the question of dependencies. These were people whose dependencies were well-satisfied, and one could work from this aspect of the individual to see how these various needs were satisfied in a large community.

(*Social process*: Fulfillment of needs and community integration can conflict.)

Langner: These (needs) have to be fulfilled now, and this is what the ideal, integrated community would be; it would be something in line with their needs. What we've been saying is that, at least for the time being, maybe 80% of our society is in an integrated set-up. Certainly for newcomers, low income groups, and so on this is not true at all; this does not fulfill their needs. The question is: Can they be integrated with a minimum of conflict for themselves, i.e., a mental strain that is minimal for mental disorientation. A curvilinear relationship might also exist between integration, especially if it's someone else's idea of rules for living. If you're integrated into this too much, you will suffer. This is what you suggested.

Brewster Smith has written about optima of mental health. You can take his ideas and say: integration of the individual can lead to incapacitation. That is, if my ideas are so much out of line with those of society, I will be considered ill according to an optima, because this has to be at an optimal level. At the same time you've got to be adjusted, there's another continuum of adjustment. Smith throws in reality orientation, too, and seemingly that is one of the problems here: the problem of sociology with functionalism, functional for whom? Everybody's been saying that someone is going to get pinched or squeezed. Dr. Chein says, "What gets in his way?"

(Editor's note: Does Henry A. Murray's TAT approach suggest also the need for a social TAT and the need for the study of the congruence of social and psychological needs? It would certainly be interesting to have a TAT profile of subjects in Stirling County.)

9. CUSTOMARY PATTERN INTERFERENCE

Whyte points out that changes in customary patterns of interaction can be another type of disintegration. Whyte (Seminar 1, pp. 34-35) observed:

(*Social process*: It's not just amount of interaction, but changes in amount.)

Whyte: It seems to me the problem is that so far we have statistical correlations between certain socio-economic conditions and the incidence of mental illness. You are trying to move from that toward sorting out the process, not toward more correlations. I want to suggest that by the time he reaches maturity, the individual has developed a certain customary pattern of interaction, and substantial changes in this pattern could lead to mental health problems, problems that could be avoided if he were able to re-establish this pattern. We should not be surprised to find an individual who has led a quite isolated life being relatively symptom-free, but we should expect that when an individual who has been involved in very active social relationships is cut off from these interactions, mental health problems of some kind will be brought on. I think it is not just a matter of how much interaction, but how it changes over time. You have to think of rewards or penalties that would occur. In brief, one way of looking at this problem is through examination of the interaction problem with particular emphasis on changes through time.

(Editor's note: Whyte's view suggests the importance of interaction process analysis for the study of social processes and mental illness, e.g., the work of Chapple, E. et al. Interaction chronograph method for analysis of differences between schizophrenics and controls, *Archives of General Psychiatry*, August, 1960, *3*, 160-167. Also, I would urge consideration of the conceptual tools of exchange theory, e.g., Thibaut, J., & Kelly, H. *The social psychology of small groups*. New York: Wiley and Sons, 1959.)

10. RESOURCE DEPRIVATION

It is clear that some people live in disorganized communities but are able to do reasonably well. Why? It may be that resource availability or resource deprivation would help account for differential adaptations. Whyte's (Seminar 1, pp. 28-29) observations are very relevant to this point.

(*Social process*: Need to account for differential response to disorganized community.)

Whyte: It seems to me that in order to test this we need to do something like this. There has been a lot of work in this Program to characterize a disorganized community, and then a lot of work on response of individuals, the symptoms that arise, and so on. What is apparently lacking is some kind of charting of the way the individual finds his way through this community. It may be that when you get this gross picture of a disorganized community, you can predict that there's a higher hazard, that succumbing to mental illnesses is higher, as in a plant where the chances are that somebody working on a dangerous job is more likely to be injured than somebody sitting at a desk. Somehow there's a differential response to this community situation. It seems to me that research has to find some method for charting the way individuals find themselves through this community so that some individuals in an over-all disorganized community, if you characterize it so, still find some kind of stable pattern of social adjustment in it, whereas others are completely lost. Apparently you are at the point where you can roughly predict, in this kind of community, that the chances of the inhabitant breaking down are greater than in another kind of community. But can you follow the individuals who do and do not break down and see how they handle it?

(*Social process*: Must consider different capacities of individuals in disorganization.)

Whyte (Seminar 1, pp. 20-21): I think there is something left out there that is important. I would like to get data on how the individual perceives the world, his attitudes, values, and so on. If we are talking about a system of relationships among people, I think we ought to look at the capacities of individuals to interact in certain patterns with others. It seems to me that it is quite a different problem that A and B face as members of the same group if, assuming the group breaks up, A is an individual who had a leadership position in this group and has been accustomed to initiating activities with a number of people. If there is not something blocking him from acting in this fashion, he may make a ready adjustment to other groups. But B is an individual who has been accustomed to being on the receiving end on social initiative; he responds, he is a follower, he may be in fine shape as long as the group is there and he is being told what to do. If the group breaks up, then we may find somebody having to counsel him: "Well, form a relationship with another group, go out and take the initiative." It may be that his interaction pattern, which has crystallized over the years, is such that he'll be in trouble until some individual or individuals take hold of him and bring him in.

So A and B could be in the same group, but their mental health problems, potentially, assuming the groups break up, would be quite different, and not just because their values, attitudes, and perceptions would be different. They might have the same goals in life, but if A can interact in a certain way and B cannot, then a breakup of the group will face them with vastly different situations.

11. INTEGRATION AND NUMBERS

The relative involvement in group memberships is an often used dimension of integration-disintegration. Yet an isolate may be doing well until pushed into personal relationships. Hodgden (Seminar 2, pp. 1-2) observed:

Hodgden: I think one could even hypothesize a situation where an individual who had been an isolate, and who for some reason had been forced or pushed into organizational patterns, might react as strongly as the person who was in a reverse situation. For example an isolate, or a slightly schizoid individual, who was drafted into the service could have a very violent reaction to this transfer into an organization.

12. SOCIAL DISCONTINUITIES

The broad range of phenomena known as social and cultural discontinuities can constitute another type of disintegration. The following seminar discussion (Seminar 2, pp. 8-18) of discontinuities is worthy of quotation in full.

(*Focus on individual*: The gang member, incapable of functioning elsewhere when it disbands, turns to narcotics to cope with the disruption.)

Chein: Let me cite an example. We think we have found in our work on narcotics with adolescents in teenage gangs that, from the point of view of an individual, the critical point, with regard to the use of narcotics, came when the gang was getting ready to break up, where the more stable individuals were making the transition from adolescence to maturity. They were establishing permanent relationships with individuals. They were beginning to establish a career line or a long-range commitment in a job, or what not. At this point, the normal pattern of gang activities is in fact disruptive; from the point of view of the gang, the fact that there are other things pulling gang members away from the gang is pathologic. From the point of view of growth of individuals, we would say it's a good thing people have to outgrow this adolescent state.

Now, the members of the gang who were unprepared for the adult role could not disband this easily. They had not laid a foundation for moving out and moving away. Their entire investment was in the gang. This was where they got their security. This is where they had their outlets. This is where they gave expression to their dependencies. Their whole life had become integrated in the functioning of the gang, and so they had an enormous investment in it.

Now, the gang is threatening to break up, and these individuals are suddenly confronted with a demand that says to them "now be a man." At this point they are incapable of functioning, and there happens to be a convenient way for them to be able to postpone that switch in their relationships, in their status, and what not, and in addition a means of preserving at least a sense of having a place in a gang, and so they become part of the drug-using class.

(*Focus on individual*: Were gang leaders better able to make other relationships than gang followers?)

Whyte: Let me put it in my own framework and see if it makes sense. I would interpret you to be saying that there was a difference in the reactions of leaders and followers in the gang. I presume those who made adjustments outside and were able to leave the gang were probably those who had had more dominant positions in the gang; they had been initiating the activities.

Chein: They did not have to follow that pattern because in the gang they might be leaders. What was crucial was that their lives were integrated around the gang.

Whyte: It would be my hypothesis from what you were saying that those who initiated activities in the gang, who were leaders, were also those who had more ties in the outside world, who had more facility for making other relationships. They could move out of the gang, and the breakup of the gang would not be traumatic for them, whereas the followers, those who had fitted into these activities in subordinate positions, found themselves high and dry without the social abilities to find other relationships.

(*Focus on individual*: Gang leadership or followership not crucial determinant for drug use, but rather degree of involvement in gang and lack of capacity to make adult commitments.)

Chein: What I'm trying to say is that it's not a leadership-fellowship condition. You could have gang members who were essentially peripheral gang members, they never developed an investment in the gang. This was a place to hang out with a group of people; this wasn't what they were dependent on, what really mattered with them. They played the role of followers because they had no real investment in this gang, there was nothing the gang was doing for them that was important, and so they didn't have to stir the gang in any special way. They were willing to go along.

On the other hand, you could have individuals who were very much involved in the gang leadership, and exactly because of their involvement in the gang leadership they drew all of their sustenance from the gang life. When other people started to depart, and the departure, you know, is not an overnight departure, they suddenly found themselves with the one thing on which their whole lives were centered vanishing, and so they turned to something else. In that process, they also lost leadership. Those who had leadership in the gang who became drug users, as the gang was approaching this splitting up, actually lost their leadership role because the user is not functional in the gang. He's a source of trouble, and the other people started to withdraw from him, to take away any attribution of leadership, and so they became isolated. They had only each other to fall back upon, other drug users, and they became involved with their connection with drugs, and the whole life that's involved in being a narcotic addict.

And now they acquired an identity, they acquired a new set of commitments because they've got things to do now, not in the short-range, but they've got long-range activities. Where other people had to be sure that they'll be able to eat next week, these guys had to be sure that they were going to be able to get their shots next week. Therefore, they had to establish a pattern of relationships within which they could get the psychological sustenance, which I take it is actually what one gets from long-range commitments.

Whyte: It would seem that the person with a leadership role, as the gang breaks up, would have more facility for establishing relationships outside, for building up new group ties, whereas the followers in the groups that I've seen appear to have a much more restrictive social orbit. Even though all the members consider themselves as being in the same gang, if you look at the patterns of interaction of each member, as far as their follower and leadership positions, those in leadership positions have a lot more interactions outside the gang than those in follower positions. I don't know that this would always happen to be true.

Hodgsen: I think this is something that could go either way, depending on the external situation beyond the gangs, and also on the personalities of the individuals in them; therefore, you wouldn't want to say the leaders always go this way and the followers always go that way.

Chein: You get gang leaders who are highly efficient and respected individuals. I remember one who got on the radio, he was terrific and was talking to a board of experts. He was a highly organized person who was able to reach out into other areas, but you also get gang leaders who are not highly organized instigators of activities. One would think of this as a leadership function. The instigators of activities are not necessarily individuals highly integrated into the surrounding world or necessarily capable of it; in this case you can have gang leaders to whom the threat of the break-up of the gang becomes something that is essentially pathogenic.

Harding: Actually, there is a good example in that very gang because there was really a rival leader, called "Holly," who was a specialist in street fighting. He was also a very smooth-talking character and quite a psychopath. Although his contacts with adults outside the gang were probably even more numerous than Harvey's (the other leader), when they were with a different type of individual, he was much more the con man. When this gang broke up it became a real problem as to where Holly would find a place in the world; he was not in very great demand as an operator in the rackets because of his street fighting propensities, and he was getting a little old for that type of thing. I never did find out what happened to him.

Whyte: Let's sum it up this way: In case the gang breaks up, who are the people who are going to have serious adjustment problems? I think on the surface this is much too simple, but maybe we might have two classes of leaders and two classes of followers roughly in terms of the interactions outside (Figure 1).

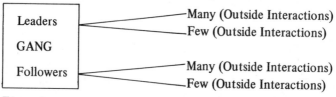

Figure 1

Here you have the sort of individual who, in spite of the fact that he has many activities within the group, also has many ties outside. I would guess, given a breakup of the group, he's going to adjust better than this fellow who has few outside ties.

By the same token, you speak of the investment a follower may have in the group; you say somebody is sort of a peripheral member. That to me means that maybe he has some leadership ability, but he may not be with the group very much. He can not gain influence in the group unless he is with them quite a bit. Perhaps followers who are more or less part of the group, but have ties outside, given a breakup of the group, will make a pretty good adjustment. Whereas, maybe it is this other type that I was suggesting earlier, who have few ties outside. When the group collapses, they have had it, there's no place for them to go. I don't know whether this fits with your observations in relation to drug addicts.

(*Focus on individual*: Gang drug user has need structure that can't be developed outside gang.)

Chein: Basically, you're right. I don't think he has to start by having narcotics. He has to have the kind of need structure that can't be developed outside. Let me take a case. Most of the kids who tend to use narcotics tend to be quite inadequate as men. In effect, insofar as they have a sex life, it is contingent on the group; other people are working things out for them, and they may participate in a line-up periodically. The other kids are not limited this way; they've got the capacity for the development of heterosexual interests, and as they start moving into a phase, whether it's biological or social (personally, I think it's social but other people think it's biological), they become interested in girls. They're able to pursue the girls, and these are not the girls necessarily who have become the ladies' auxiliary of the gang. They've got the capacity to move away from the gang, and as their interests pull them away, they move; they don't have to start with the outside contacts. I think the reasonable hypothesis is that the guys who have these capacities are also likely to exercise them.

(*Focus on individual*: Doubtful that individual dependent on others for social activity; able to initiate others if customary ones disappear.)

Whyte: My guess would be that you develop something in your social security that has to do with good social relationships. I do not know if there is anything inherent in the individual that predisposes him one way or the other, but I would be surprised if an individual who has never initiated social activity, who has always been dependent upon the efforts of others and finds himself in a situation where these customary ties are gone, with nobody else taking him in, would be going out and establishing himself in these relationships.

(*Focus on individual*: Dissolution an advantage in adjustment; Chein—capacity to reach out crucial.)

A. Leighton: You have emphasized that the person having outside contacts at the time the boundaries of the gang dissolve has an advantage then in hooking on to something else. Dr. Chein has emphasized the resources of the individual, saying, even if he did not have those hooks at the time the gang dissolved, some people have the capacity to reach out and establish it at that critical time and others don't.
Whyte: I am assuming that the capacity to do so grows out of some kind of experience in having done so.

(*Focus on individual*: People have capacities for leadership in some situations, not necessarily because of prior experience.)

A. Leighton: Summarizing what you both said, somewhat inadequately, but to lay a basis for a third point that I think is worth weighing into this, there are characteristic situations that either your leader or your follower can meet, and other characteristic situations that they cannot function in so well. Edna Ferber's novel *Cimarron* is about a man who is marvelous in the frontier situation but could not function once it had become a stable society. He became a bum until he moved to a new frontier, and then he would rise to the top again. Barrie's play, *The admirable crichton*, is about a fellow who was a butler; he got wrecked on a desert island and became the Emperor. When he was rescued from the desert island and he went back to civilization, he became a butler once again. Tyhurst has a dramatic account of a fire that broke out in Halifax in a department store. There had been in this department store for a number of years a mousy switchboard operator, as I remember it, a maiden lady in her 40's who had never done much or said much; one of those vegetable types, reflecting the type of background that she had before. When a fire broke out and everybody began running around, the bells were ringing and so on, she started calling up people all over the store, telling them what to do; telling them to shut the windows to keep drafts from coming in and increasing the fire; telling the elevator people to close the elevators; telling people to go to the stairs and control the crowd; directing, telephoning outside and calling the police and the fire department; and she called everybody from the manager down to the front door porter, all from the switchboard and told them what they should do in this crisis, and they all did it. They were all wondering what to do, and when somebody said "do this, do that" they did it, and so in this half-hour or hour, in this crisis of a fire, she ran the department store, and then subsided again.

I think part of the problem is that people have capacities for being leaders in some kind of contact, and not in others. Just as an example of this, some people do well as leaders in strategic situations. They are not good at tactics. If they have a chance to plan long-range, or medium-range, what's to be done, they do it pretty well; but if they have to decide now, among a whole lot of differential distinctions they don't do it very well. And there are other people who can decide in a practical situation, with a whole lot of things hitting them now; when they have got to decide right away, they can decide pretty well, but they don't have the capacity for long-range planning. Some people can do both. This is one temperamental variation, and there may be others.

Another variation is the type of person who can function quite well in a leadership role as long as he's got the kind of structure in a social system that you have in a military unit. He can function in a military unit, Boy Scouts unit, or a civil service bureau, but there's the other kind of leader who can function in a fluid situation, as in politics where there is a mixture of pressures and persuasions and balancing things against the other, yet who would be very badly off in a highly structured military situation.

This kind of difference strikes me because, from the point of view of treating patients, every once in a while if you see strongly into the dynamics of the patient, you see he's really the kind of a person who has leadership capacities, but this structure has dissolved and the medium he now finds himself in is one in which he can't exercise those particular talents. They are not transferable to that situation, but having another situation which was analogous to the one he just left, he might be able to transfer them to it.

(Editor's note: Maybe we need a more systematic way of charting and classifying role processes over time, as for example, the above case of shifting patterns of superordination-subordination).

13. POOR ROLE-PERSONALITY ALLOCATION

Another type of disintegration is the discrepancy between role demands and personality types. Chein referred to poor career channeling within an organization as a possible example of this problem. For example, the channels for advancement in an organization can determine the proper or improper use of an individual's capacities.

The following brief conversation (Seminar 2, pp. 19-20) is instructive:

(*Focus on social units*: Channels for advancement in organization can determine proper or improper use of individual's capacities.)

Chein: We can take the channels that social organizations offer for advancement, as, for example, the group workers. This is a field in which the basic training of the people is for one level of work. They are highly sensitive to functioning in small groups. They can fit into it, they can facilitate the operation, encouraging the youngsters to develop, etc. It is a relatively new profession so vertical mobility is very rapid.

For example, you get somebody who graduates from the New York School of Social Work, and in a few years he's the assistant head of a large agency. He has moved now into a new level of responsibility for which he is totally unequipped. Everything that he has ever learned about group work may suddenly vanish, and then he becomes a tyrant, unreasonable, petty, all kinds of things that he would never be if he were functioning as group worker.

Now, as administrators, such people have a completely new set of challenges, and basically what I would say about this profession is that its structure is haywire because there should be channels for advancement within the level of skills of the individuals, of what it is that they are capable of and best equipped to do. Instead, this professional structure is one that does something quite different. This is true of the academic profession. Once you've reached the stage of a full professor, the only way you can advance is to move into administration, and if the financial rewards, or the status rewards, are important to you, here's the situation. Hence, you end up doing the things that you're least equipped to do, that you don't want to do, that you're not organized to do.

Whyte: This is true of an awful lot of professions. Your engineer starts out with emphasis on his technical skills and later on you hear nobody taught him anything about administration. It's a fairly common problem.

Chein: I think so but this is what I take to be an example of a bad social organization. It is essentially a disintegrated pattern within the way society is organized. It puts individuals into situations, and rewards them for situations in which they are inadequate to function.

The foregoing represents a range of views on how social processes can be disintegrative or interfering. Throughout the foregoing comments this question is posed: What is the nature of a healthy social system?

In the process of the seminar, several attempts were made to summarize the integration-disintegration concept. One summary statement consists of a conversation by Raymond Illsley, Alexander H. Leighton, Jane Murphy, William Foote Whyte, and John Harding; a second summary is by Raymond Illsley; a third is a statement by Isidor Chein (Seminar 2, pp. 73-74); and finally a summary by Alexander Leighton.

Summary 1. Conversation by Raymond Illsley, Alexander H. Leighton, John Harding, Jane Murphy, and William F. Whyte

(*Social process*: Integration-disintegration being used in many ways, and interchangeably with organization-disorganization, urgent to look at concept.)

Illsley: Looking through the documents after the meeting, I was really struck by the way in which we were all using integration in different senses, and I listed some of the ways in which this had been used. On the one hand, there was some talk of the integration of an individual into a community. There was just one reference to this particular problem.

Then there was much more discussion about integration between an individual's values, sentiments, and so on, and the situation in which he found himself. I, myself, was thinking very much more in terms of the integration of a person's social network: how far people with whom he interacts are people who know each other, who meet each other; how far the whole network of acquaintance is an integrated one. Then, we came across the idea of integration-disintegration of a community, or of a group.

I personally would even like to discuss the difference between whether we really mean disintegration, or whether we mean non-integration, disintegration, rather, assuming that there had previously been integration. We tend, I think, too, to use the terms "social disintegration," and "social disorganization" as being the same thing, whereas perhaps they aren't the same thing. I wouldn't say that integration was the same as organization even if the two opposites were concerned.

Dr. Chein not long ago said that if he were to have a new integration, this for him would mean having a new personality. These are all different senses it seems to me in which we're using these words, and I have the feeling we have got to get together in order to look at this conception, perhaps in relation to one problem.

(Social process: Need for dictionary of term "integration" to clarify concept and help group's communication.)

A. Leighton: I feel strongly about what you have just said. Perhaps in between one of these Seminars, fairly soon, in cooperation with you, Dr. Freydberg, or Dr. Murphy, we should really work out a sort of dictionary of the term "integration" so that we could have this as something to which we could refer. It was really the contribution by Kluckholm and Kroeber on the use of the word "culture" that was of help in clarifying this concept. It was used with something like 150 different meanings and was confusing to everybody who tried to talk about it when they were using it in different ways. I think this would be a really substantial contribution to the progress of communications in this group, and perhaps for other people too, to get this cleared up.

(Focus: Either should investigate environment noxious to individual or meaning of disintegration of social systems going back and forth showing diminishing returns.)

We're really facing though, aside from that, a decision that we'd better make. It came up last time and it's here again. That is, whether we should continue to build up along the line that Dr. Chein outlined: define the kind of social environment that is noxious to the individual; after we've got this mapped out, when everybody has thought about it and made contributions to the progress of communications in this group, and perhaps for other people too, we'll have this cleared up.

Through this, perhaps, then we can work ourselves back into integration and disintegration. We may also do what Harding says, which is to turn the thing around and say, here are people who've worked in different kinds of social systems, let's see if we can define what is meant by disintegration of a social system or, conversely, integration of a social system, using as the examples Whyte's experience in organization and other experience that people here have had with social systems. This is what I think Hinkle was advocating last time, and after we have defined integration as a social problem, not as a psychological problem that makes systems function or not function, nor as the components that make for a functionally effective system or not, then we can move back again from that to say what the effects of this kind of a system are on the development of the individual.

As was pointed out in the first Seminar, it probably doesn't matter too much which of these places you begin with if you're going to go from one to the other eventually. You're going to do both, but as John has just said, I think we are reaching the point of diminishing returns in trying to do the two simultaneously; therefore, I think we probably ought to have some kind of focus, right now. I'd like to propose that we pursue one or the other.

Murphy: I agree but would like to make one point before we go on. In considering the integration-disintegration of a social system, it's possible to think of it as being what you see happening at just one point in time. This is mainly what we have been doing in our community studies in Nova Scotia. It has struck me as I listened to these various ideas about integration-disintegration within a gang or within an organization that we are injecting a very valuable component—longevity. We have been talking about the switch from an adolescent gang orientation to a more mature life pattern. We've talked about mobility upward in a professional organization where certain conflicts occur at certain points. These are clearly not matters of looking at the environment at just one time. They point out that there may be disintegrative crisis points or integrative crisis points in the total history of an environmental unit.

(*Social process*: Definitional clarity of integration-disintegration.)

Whyte: I think that what has been lacking so far is anything but a correlation study between integrated and disintegrated communities and a certain prevalence of mental illness. Now, I would like the definition of integration-disintegration, which has been crude, to be improved upon, but if that is going to be especially productive, it seems to me that the research strategy has to have the time dimension emphasized more. For example, you might follow certain individuals through time, partly retrospectively, trace out their maneuverings in their various social spheres, and hopefully partly following them in the present and in the future in their work with organizations, groups, associations—however you can get a base of a number of interacting individuals. Then you have a kind of research that would follow that social unit through time to observe the changes, and to see what kind of effect these changes have upon individuals.

It seems to me that unless there's some way of getting the time relation into the research, you remain on this correlational level; a disintegrated community defined in more precise terms would show that you would have more problems with mental illness, but just what is the social process that makes it come out this way; you can't get at it without some longitudinal effort.

(*Social process*: One Nova Scotia community has changed from disintegrated to integrated, and plans exist to make changes with predicted effects.)

A. Leighton: I've worked with this emphasis on time, and this is very congenial to us. We have one instance of a community that was disintegrated 10 years ago that has now changed into an integrated community, and where we have taken a sociological, psychological, and psychiatric resurvey. We have tremendously ambitious plans in prospect for trying deliberately to change communities and predict what the effect will be. Whether we can pull this off or not, I don't know.

Harding: It seems to me that a longitudinal type of approach is essential, but it seems to me that it is most fruitful if it can be organized around the notion of asking what it is that's changing over time, or what different things are changing. The simplest, almost crudest way, of putting the question is to say, to give an example, if there is a change, let's say induced by some external forces, that leads to a change in the integration of one particular small community, do we find an accompanying change over time in the average mental health status in the population there, or don't we?

The opposite way of doing it is: If we introduce a rush of people of lower mental health status in the community, if we could help them in there, would we find that the level of community integration went down if we looked at it over time?

Well, this is merely speculative, but in any event it seems to me that this kind of thinking is illustrative of the value of focusing the examination of concrete social processes and structures, and the changes in them around a variable or set of variables. At the same time, you should be asking yourself just what is it that is changing, and do we actually mean the same thing when we say that a community becomes more disintegrated over a 1 to 2 year period as we mean when we say that the adolescent gang disintegrates or becomes disintegrated in time?

Is it the same thing that we mean when we say that a community becomes more disintegrated, and if it isn't exactly the same thing, how is it different?

2. Illsley's Summary Observations

What I have to say on this stems from some of our earlier remarks about integration. I was the one who was a little confused about the way the term "integration" was being used and began to have a look at these. One particular definition of this word is closely linked to the kind of ideas that are set out in the second paragraph of the agenda about this interlinking of social and kinship networks. I began to look at the degree to which a person's community of interest, his patterns of interactions, were integrated together, or whether they took a more diffuse form. I was thinking particularly of the difference between small communities, as you get in Nova Scotia or Northern Scotland, and the kind of community you might get in midtown Manhattan. I got one or two profiles of people's lives and worked them out in the following way: I took people living in a very restricted community and looked at the various groups with which they mixed, such as their extended family, their neighbors, their work colleagues, their work colleagues' families, various interest groups that they might be associated with in the community, either political, recreational, and so on, and then whole sets of what you might call friendship clusters. (See Figure 2.)

I set out along one axis each of these different groups, and put the same block down the other axis, and began by having a look at the extent to which each of these groups with whom the person mixed, interrelated, were residents in the same locality, in the small community, and in the working class area in a larger city, the total network of acquaintances was wholly within the geographical community. They had no acquaintances outside. When I look at whether one

	family	extended family	neighbors	work colleagues	work colleagues' families	religious groups	political groups	recreational groups
family		yes	yes	no	no	yes	no	yes
extended family			no	no	no	yes	no	no
neighbors				no	no	no	yes	yes
work colleagues					yes	no	yes	no
work colleagues' families						no	no	no
religious groups*							no	no
political groups*								no
recreational groups*								

*Each separate one would be listed

Figure 2. Profile of interpersonal systems.

Note: This matrix can help to determine the extent to which the various systems are interrelated or separate. For example, whether one's family and one's work colleagues' families intermingle, etc.

group with whom they mixed knew another group, again I found that in the small community you got integration in the sense that a person's network was indeed a network in that they interacted with people all around them, and these people were, at the same time, in eracting with all other members whom they knew.

(*Focus on the individual—Environment*: The groups to which an individual belongs in a small community are likely to intermingle geographically as well as socially. This is less likely in large communities where groups of interest may be scattered and the geographical factor is of less meaning.)

When you came, however, to look at two other examples, people living in larger cities and people living in a professional group, you found a very different kind of situation, in that, as you looked at their various groups, you'd find that a smaller and smaller proportion of them existed within their geographical community. Not only this, you'd find that what groups they were acquainted with, were not necessarily acquainted with each other, so that they stand at the center of a network in which they knew the people out here on the periphery, but the people on the periphery did not know each other.

This was a network of which they were the center, but it wasn't as set as it was in bilateral arrangements. It seemed to me that this is very much the kind of difference that you're likely to get when you move over from the study of a larger community to the study of a smaller community, and also, I think, the kind of difference you'll get if you look at a group that is highly migrant, as professional groups, and a group that is more static, particularly the unskilled working groups.

This notion reminded me of some of the work that had been done by an anthropologist, Elizabeth Bott, and reported in her book, *Family and Social Networks*, in which she looked at some 25 families in London in great detail, actually living in the home for hours on end.

She looked at their kind of networks, too, and she found very marked differences in other characteristics of people who had networks of a different kind. She was particularly interested in marital role segregation, and on this relatively small but highly static sample she found that where you had a pattern of relationships that were not integrated, you tend to get more joint roles, less segregation. Where you got the other type of network, then here you tended to have highly segregated roles between husbands and wives.

She looked at many factors in this situation and some of them could be explained, one kind of class, one kind of merit pattern, and also one kind of family and/or social relationships. There seemed to be some in the lower group that were not dependent on class, age, and things of this kind. I felt that this was the kind of idea that we might discuss; we might particularly discuss it too, not only with regard to the notion of integration, but also with regard to the notion of community. When you're dealing with these different kinds of networks, if you can sufficiently systematize them, you can begin to work out along this line what a person's community is. It may be very simple in a small village, their geographical community is identical with their set of social and kinship relations.

3. Chein's Summary Observations

I've been making some jottings during the meeting and I have a little contribution to make in terms of integration-disintegration. A social group or social context, or social what-have-you is integrated to the degree in which (a) the individuals involved are facilitated in carrying on with the major activities to which they are committed and the activities that are expected of them, and find their personal commitments congruent with what is expected of them; and (b) the dialectics of change are such that the transformations in commitments and/or expectations that are consequent upon such carryings on or

upon the maturation of the individuals involved will not disrupt the
balance described in (a).

(*Rationale for definition of integration*: People are involved in activities
because they want to be and it's expected of them. Doing these things
requires support. Changes occur and they must be absorbed with
harmony.)

What I tried to put into this is the notion that people are involved in
activities. They're involved in activities because they want to be
involved in activities, because these are things that are expected of
them, and there's a potential source of disintegration in defects and
impatience. Secondly, I put into this the fact that doing things requires
support; we can't operate if there's a possibility of disruption
emanating from the failure to provide a space dimension of facilitation.
And I put into it the notion that things don't remain the same.
Consequently, the changes that occur, if these are changes that lead
into it progressively from the point of view of facilitation and harmony
within the ranks, then the expectation is for a well-integrated situation.
If from this point of view the situation progressively deteriorates,
because successive outcomes lead into situations that are no longer
compatible with the harmony of either the supports or the activities,
the two sources of the activity, this is a bad situation, and from a
temporary point of view, this is not a well-integrated situation.

Summary View 4: "Some Notes on the Concept
of Disintegration,"
by Alexander H. Leighton, M.D.

Any system by definition involves integration. Integration is part of
the condition of being a system. When a system changes toward
disintegration it is moving away from being a system. At absolute

disintegration, the system no longer exists, although its component parts may continue. A cell, a whole animal, a hive of bees, a community, an orchestra, a ship's crew, an army, are examples.

Systems perform functions. This is what is meant by dynamic. It follows therefore that as a system changes in the direction of disintegration, its functions also change in the direction of nonexistence. Life is threatened, economic acitivity depreciates, music is badly produced, the ship is late, the army bungles, etc. Disintegration is not the sole possible cause of malfunction, and one can see at times sufficient functioning in the face of some disintegration. This is because a system can often bring compensatory factors into play, or the disintegration may be localized within the system. In the long run, however, disintegration adversely affects function and at absolute disintegration all functioning has ceased.

The Stirling County and Yoruba projects attempted to check the hypothesis that socio-cultural disintegration causes psychiatric disorders. Cast in such general terms, however, this hypothesis can be misleading. It is important to indicate, therefore, that its point of reference is exclusively the small community. What it actually says is that the small community is a system such that the greater the disintegration, the greater the failure in community functions and the greater this malfunctioning, the more adverse the effect on the mental health of the members. The community is looked upon as a quasi-organism—an energy system with fairly discrete boundaries and with human components who exercise most aspects of their lives within the system.

It is important to recognize the limits of the concept and hypothesis. They do not say, for instance, that general cultural disintegration produces psychiatric disorder. In the first place, culture is an abstraction that refers to aspects of many communities and not wholly to any one. In the second place, a culture may disintegrate and even disappear while the communities affected may continue without much disintegration by developing or adopting a new culture. It is possible, however, to extend the concepts of disintegration beyond the village base that has been employed in the Stirling and Yoruba Studies. There is no reason that it cannot be applied to much larger units such as cities and even nations. But emphasis must be given the word "unit." The point of reference has to be in some sense a society—a community of inter-dependent people, a system with definable margins. Thus one could, if the operational criteria be found, compare London and New York, or Nigeria and the Congo. That is to say each of these could as systems be compared with regard to their relative degree of integration. Further, according to the hypothesis, wide discrepancies of integration between them would be accompanied by wide differences in mental health.

From the point of view of advancing knowledge regarding the relationship of socio-cultural factors and mental health, there are difficulties in attempting to compare such large units. At the practical level there are problems of the cost and personnel that would be required to gather the multitude of necessary data. But even if this were feasible, it remains doubtful that the establishment of such global relationships would bring us much closer to establishing which specific socio-cultural factors affect mental health and especially how they do it.

It is possible for a part of a system to be disintegrated. That is to say, a subsystem within a system may be to a conspicuous degree disintegrated and malfunctional without this applying to the system as a whole. It is thus theoretically possible to compare at least certain subsystems within communities and between communities with regard to degree of integration and disintegration.

There are difficulties in this, however. The subsystems have to be chosen with care so they actually constitute comparable types of phenomena. Two industries in different communities might be compared, or two police forces, but not likely a police force and an industry. *Whole* systems, furthermore, cannot be compared with *parts* of other systems. The integration of a small town may not, without violation of the concept, be compared to the integration of an industry or city block, or a social class.

The hypothesis that links integration to mental health does not apply to subsystems. This is because the hypothesis is predicated on the assumption that most inhabitants of a community live most aspects of their lives there. Thus the level of integration has a widespread effect—on work, family life, growth and development, recreation, health, aspirations, sense of trust in the future, etc. Most subsystems affect only a portion of life—the working hours or recreation time, or social life, or education, etc. Thus the psychologically noxious effects of disintegration in a subsystem may be compensated or neutralized by factors at work in other parts of the system.

To repeat and summarize: While the term "disintegration" can be applied to a variety of social phenomena, the hypothesis relating it to mental health obtains only when it is applied to whole social systems—that is communities.

This brings forward the fact that it is the way the socio-cultural environment impinges on the individual that is of crucial importance. We may call this contact between the net effect of the socio-cultural environment and the experiencing individual the "interphase." The hypothesis may now be restated to say that disintegrated interphases produce psychiatric disorder. In disintegrated communities there are more disintegrated interphases than in well integrated communities.

By chance, of course, there will be some disintegrated interphases in all communities, even the best integrated. It may also be that the patterning of a community system is such that certain categories of persons experience disintegrated interphases while other categories do not. We have some evidence that in Stirling County the village of Fairhaven is experienced as integrated by the men and relatively disintegrated by the women. The converse appears to be true of La

Vallee. In many places it would seem that with advancing years, particularly between 60 and 70, a person is confronted with a progressively disintegrated interphase.

The concept of the disintegrated interphase is possibly an appropriate one with which to approach the problem of the environmental factors that affect mental health in large towns and cities. If we take the city as a community—a whole system—we can examine its patterns and structure to see if certain of the subsystems regularly have a disintegrative effect during their portion of the interphase for any considerable number of people. Certain work situations, for example, might well fall into this category. We can then see if there are certain roles or categories of persons that regularly constitute totally disintegrative interphases because of the way they are linked to several disintegrated subsystems. Thus the man who experiences a disintegrated work situation, a disintegrated housing situation, and an impoverished religious, social, and recreational life may be regarded as living in a disintegrated environment, even though the city as a whole or even most of its subsystems may not be properly so regarded.

The problem, then, becomes one of examining the socio-cultural patterning and functioning of the city to see where large numbers of disintegrative interphases are being produced. These must be definable, of course, by objective criteria that are independent of the criteria used for estimating the presence or absence of psychiatric disorder. When such have been defined and tested they can then be used to explore the hypothesis that relate them to mental health.

It is clear that a variety of ways of looking at the concepts of integration-disintegration were expressed in the seminar. It is also apparent that a complex range of important phenomena are suggested by these terms.

In a historical sense, the concept of integration has had a long and interesting history from Durkheim on through to such scholars as

Landecker, Angell, Wirth, Parsons, Bales, Odum, and many others. In a seminar held by the Social Science Research Council in the early 1950s, Robin Williams found that integration had been defined to include the following, and this was not meant as an exhaustive list [2]:

1. Smooth functioning, e.g. the absence of conflict; closely coordinated behaviors
2. The attractiveness of a group or society to its members, e.g., the unwillingness to leave, willingness to make sacrifices to retain membership, feelings of belonging
3. Pattern-consistency of cultural elements; logical meaningful integration; cultural integration; ethos
4. Consensus on norms for behavior
5. Conformity with norms
6. Communicative integration; extent and kind of exchange of meanings among persons within the unit or system
7. Functional interdependence; economic, political, or other "ecological" linkage
8. Capacity for concerted action to meet external threat or other crisis
9. Absence of psychological distress or "mental illness" among individuals in the grouping
10. Social predictability; the certainty and clarity of expectations

To my knowledge, Alexander H. Leighton's *My Name is Legion* [3] is the most recent and most systematic attempt to synthesize an empirically relevant theory of integration-disintegration. As indicated, this book develops the frame of reference for the Stirling County Study. And the results of this study have brought us back again to a reassessment of the concepts of integration-disintegration.

At this point, John French's assessment of the theory of integration-

[2] Williams, Robin Jr. Unity and diversity in modern America. *Social Forces*, October 1957, *36*, 1-8.
[3] Leighton, Alexander H. *My name is legion*. New York: Basic Books, 1959.

disintegration may prove very stimulating to our concern with clarifying these concepts (Seminar 11, p. 2-22).

French: Maybe I should say that in reading over the previous seminar notes and your original proposal, I find much that I agree with. Furthermore, many of my reactions have already been stated by others. I think it might be most helpful if I would quickly skip over all the areas in which I'm delighted to find that we're working on the same problems and approaching them in the same way. So I'll try to pick out those places where I think maybe we would have a difference of approach, or opinion, or idea. Of course, negative criticism is so easy in this difficult area of mental health that I'd like to try to restrict myself with the following comment: Wherever I have a criticism, I think I shouldn't mention it, unless I think I know what ought to be done about it. You are going to see that I am always overreaching myself. But I would be glad to crawl out on the limb and let you saw it off.

Now, there are three kinds of comments that I have.

First, a lot of the differences, as you might expect, really stem from one's philosophy of a science, from metatheoretical conceptions, from purposes, from general strategic conceptions of research. Second, we can narrow down to a set of theoretical questions. This might be where we should spend the most time, and especially in the area of status, which is of interest to you, of interest to me, and of interest to the project. Third, I have a few reactions to methodological issues.

Well, let me then present, not all, but a sampling, of some of the more likely useful ones. I'll start with a couple of rather broad metatheoretical points, because that will most quickly show up the source of my biases. And then we'll go on to some of the more theoretical issues where it might be more useful to have a discussion.

I think the first and most general comment that I had concerns the remarks I read about the environment—I'm talking now about your purposes to study the effects of the environment on mental health and to develop conceptual clarity about your two key variables of status and disintegration.

Now, let me see if I can state a little bit more about what I think some of the problems were, and some solutions. I'll do this briefly. Then, if anyone wants to come back to this one item, we can.

When I read the word "environment" I never knew whether you were talking about that environment that was coming in contact with the individual person. Does it really impinge on him and affect his mental health? Surely only a tiny fraction of New York City ever impinges on any single individual; most of the metropolis never touches him. That's part of it.

Then, I began to wonder: Are you talking about the psychological environment or the objective environment? Here I will introduce my distinctions. They are presented in Figure 3 which is in both of my *Journal of Social Issues* articles [4]. This diagram is a kind of metatheoretical conception of the kinds of variables that ought to be studied in order to understand the effect of the environment on mental health.

There are two boxes for the environment. The objective environment as it exists; this includes not only the physical environment, the food or the buildings, but the social environment, the society, the culture, the social organization, and the face-to-face group. These elements are all objectively existing out there, outside the individual. The psychological environment is these elements as he perceives them; and I would include unconscious perception. (We know that he perceives unconsciously because he reacts and behaves in terms of it.) I assume that the objective environment influences mental health primarily by way of its influence on the psychological environment.

The second kind of broad question concerns research strategy. This is to say: "I think you people have learned so much already about the

[4] Work, health, and satisfaction. *Journal of Social Issues*, July, 1962, *18*, 3. The social environment and mental health. *Journal of Social Issues*, 1963, *19*, 4, Pp. 39-56.

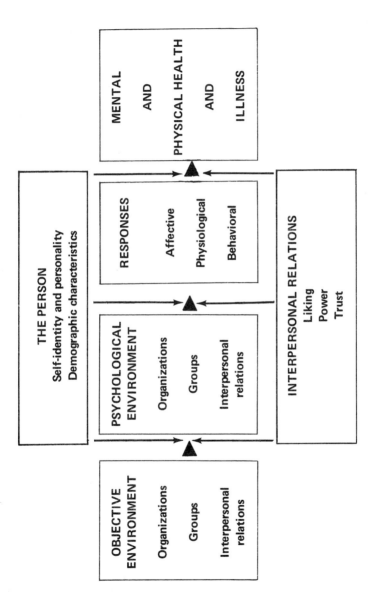

Figure 3. The six panels of variables involved in an environmental approach to mental health together with the major types of hypotheses (horizontal arrows) and conditioning variables (vertical arrows).

correlation between status and mental health, or the correlation between social integration-disintegration and mental health, that your next task should be gap-filling. You ought to ask, "Why this correlation?"

This would include what is causing what, here? Does poor mental health produce social disorganization, or vice versa? But you also ought to ask "Why?," in the sense of what are the intervening variables and mechanisms?

If we are able to say, now, it is status that is influencing mental health, we should ask by what means? Why does it do so? What are the variables that intervene? Again Figure 3 indicates that you ought to look at the psychological environment, the perceived status as the individual perceives it. But then you must also look at responses. How does he behave? How does he feel? What is his affective response? And finally, physiological responses. All of you people, I'm sure, have a much better background for studying such matters and programatically speaking, I would urge that you ought to be doing it rather than me. But all of us, I think, ought to be doing it, and I will be glad to cite some findings of mine, really more Sid Cobb's findings, that argue powerfully that we ought to try to do both at once. That, again, is a kind of general conceptual metatheoretical problem.

Now, a third thing, still in this area, that I'd like to mention: I think when we get down to trying to fill the gaps, trying to link across the objective environment-subjective environment, trying to see the person's responses to that, and what, in turn, that does to his mental health and his psychiatric illnesses, I think then we need to feel we have commensurate dimensions, commensurate concepts, commensurate measures. What I mean by this is that we can measure variables in two or more boxes on the same scale. For example, we can measure objective status and subjective status on the same scale. I raise this because I noticed you were concerned with the concept of "fit"; how does this person fit his environment? I noticed that you are interested in the very broad general question, "To what extent does the social environment fit the needs of the person?"

Well, to get specific, we would have to measure that, and conceptualize that on commensurate dimensions. If he has a need for love and affection as a person, then we need to measure how much love and affection there is in the environment. It's the affection that needs to be measured rather than how much food. But if he is suffering from starvation, let us measure the amount of food in the environment, or the supplies he gets from an environment. Only if we can measure the needs of the person and the supplies in the environment on commensurate dimensions can we derive a quantitative discrepancy score that measures the degree of person-environment fit [5].

Let's move to theory. I've been particularly interested in the development of self-concept or self-identity theory as a way to expand and help us with the social side of the person and with the personal side of the social environment.

You'll see a main theme running through my reactions to your theoretical approach. First of all, in looking at integration-disintegration, I have a feeling that you've really got hold of something important here, and I'm willing to take it as proven. Now I think you ought to be more analytical about it. This is too global a concept. It's a set of variables, and so the next step ought to be to examine them more analytically; on an unidimensional basis look into the intercorrelations of the variables within this concept. We should have hypotheses, not about integration-disintegration and its effects on mental health, but about each of the separate variables and their

[5] The concepts and methods for measuring person-environment fit are described more fully in French, J. R. P., Jr. The conceptualization and measurement of mental health in terms of self-identity theory. In S. Sells (Ed.) *The definition and measurement of mental health*, Washington, D.C.: U.S. Government Printing Office, to be published.

effects on mental health. Then, we should sometimes summate, some way or other, to see what the total effects are.

Well, that's the theme; then this would begin to get over into the measurement level. If we are thinking of the conceptual definition of integration-disintegration such as this, then what's the appropriate operational definition? And I had some feeling there were discrepancies there. With this concept you ought to be measuring something different here in New York than what you're measuring in Nova Scotia. As you move from Stirling County to Manhattan there are going to be, as you've been noting, real problems; and the problems, I think, are partly this: How global a concept is it? Do you try to operationalize it at the level of the over-all concept, or the subvariables? And are your conceptual definitions clear enough, are they abstract enough, to point specifically to how you ought to operationalize it now in a very different setting such as Manhattan?

A second theoretical suggestion would be to do the same thing with status or social class, or socio-economic status, as another concept that is too global.

Now, speaking of my own research, I have started out dealing with status and have been quite convinced that it is much too global a concept. There ought to be a law against anybody's ever using the concept of social class; there ought to be a law against anybody's stating a hypothesis about social class and mental health. They ought to be forced to deal with more analytical component variables of occupational level, income level, and educational level. They ought to be defining it abstractly enough so that they are also looking at other dimensions of social class or status. For example, if you're dealing with Negroes, you ought to look at how light or dark the skin color is. That happens to be an important dimension of status for Negroes, citing Robert Kleiner's work. I would say, if you're dealing with any community, including one in Nova Scotia, that power is a dimension of status. This gets neglected by everybody in this kind of issue.

Now, I don't take this to be a metatheoretical bias, or theoretical prejudice; I think I have good empirical evidence to prove you all ought to do this; let me mention several kinds of evidence, which I could review and talk about and discuss.

(1). There's a tremendous amount of evidence that indicates that it's not only status that's related to mental health, it's status incongruence; that means specifically, and by definition, you have to look at separate dimensions of status and see whether they are congruent with one another. How discrepant is your status in education, compared with your income?

(2). In this area I would include the husband-wife discrepancies. To give you an example, in one of our studies of rheumatoid arthritis in families, we find that rheumatoid arthritis is associated with a discrepancy in education between the husband and the wife. If the wife has more education than her husband, or vice versa, she's likely to have rheumatoid arthritis.

(3). I'm now convinced that the level of aspiration theory is a very powerful kind of theory in our society, our achieving society, for thinking about mental health, all the way from schizophrenia down to job satisfaction. And there's a lot of research there. Again, Kleiner's research in Philadelphia is the most extensive following from this; I could also cite our own research, showing how a level of aspiration theory illuminates problems of status, status incongruence, and status discrepancy between husband and wife. So, if we really want to examine that issue, maybe we ought to look at some of the data.

Kleiner studied a probability sample of 1,500 Negroes for the whole city of Philadelphia who were not hospitalized, and he had a hospital sample as well [6].

His first assumption is that in our society, the person who has a higher level of education will have a higher level of aspiration,

[6] Parker, S., & Kleiner, R. J. *Mental illness in the urban Negro community*. New York: The Free Press, 1966.

aspiration with respect to occupation and income. That's an assumption with respect to this set of studies that had never been tested previously.

He makes a second assumption that success and failure are determined by achievement above and below the level of aspiration. This assumption is supported by literally hundreds of carefully controlled laboratory experiments on the level of aspiration. If your performance is above your level of aspiration, you feel success; if it's below, you feel failure.

He makes a third assumption that this can be generalized beyond performance and feelings of success or failure with respect to a specific task. In fact, the whole self-concept is affected. Putting it in my terms, if you're a Negro, and your aspired self is to become a plumber, this would be a very high level of aspiration. But you end up becoming a garbage man. There will be a discrepancy between the aspired self and the achieved self, and consequently low self-esteem; this will be related to schizophrenia.

Now, even before Kleiner did this field survey to check directly on this, he looked to see how this would jibe with other data he had on Negroes who were educated in the South and then migrated to Philadelphia and presumably had a lower level of aspiration for occupation. You would predict a lower discrepancy: that these Negroes didn't expect to become plumbers, they only expected to become garbage men. And from this hypothesis then, you would predict better mental health, or more specifically, less prevalence of schizophrenia. However, if you take the migration hypothesis, you'd predict the opposite, migrants should have more than the natives.

Well, the data he had supported the level of aspiration hypothesis here. Migrants who were from the South had less schizophrenia than the native born; migrants from the North who were educated as Philadelphia Negroes and who should have similar levels of aspiration, were just like the natives from Philadelphia, the nonmigrants, in the incidence of schizophrenia; that would be a better way of putting it in these earlier studies.

Now, he goes on with a hospital sample and also a population sample. To test this theory, we've got to measure all the concepts involved. That is, we've got to measure their level of aspiration, for occupation, for income. We've got to measure the size of the discrepancy between what is obtained and what is aspired, and correlate that directly with the dependent mental health variables.

Now, I've left out some of the additional, intervening variables that are in the level of aspiration theory, especially when you begin to relate it to achievement theory: valence of success, valence of failure, probability of success, and probability of failure. He measured all of those to obtain the resultant valence, which is a complex function of these variables.

His results confirmed the assumptions and hypotheses that I have sketched. Higher education does lead to a higher level of aspiration with respect to occupation. Those who fail to achieve these occupational aspirations, and thus suffer a status incongruence, also experience more goal-striving stress; and they show a higher incidence of hospitalization for mental illness. The data support the interpretation that the effects of status incongruence and of goal-striving stress are mediated by lowered self-esteem. Of course, there are severe methodological problems with data on hospitalization, but these are largely avoided in this research because the same general theory was also supported by the data on severity of symptoms in the community sample.

Our own studies of status incongruence extend these findings and emphasize the importance of breaking down the global concept of status when studying mental health [7]. We find that status incongruence within a single parent and status discrepancy between the two parents produces illness in their adult offspring. Such status stress produces rheumatoid arthritis in the daughter (but not in the son),

[7] Kasl, S. V., & Cobb, S. Effects of parental status incongruence and discrepancy on physical and mental health of adult offspring. *Journal of Personal and Social Psychology*, 1967, 7 (2), Pp. 1-15.

reported poor physical health, symptoms of physical anxiety, and feelings of anxiety, anger, depression, and low self-confidence.

Finally, I mentioned to some of you some very fascinating indications that the frustrated man in our society, who does not meet his own level of aspiration with respect to occupation, i.e., suffers status incongruence with respect to education and occupation, projects it onto his firstborn son; the son accepts this, and he goes to the University of Michigan Medical School. And so we find that, compared to chance expectations, there is an excess of first-borns and a dearth of last-borns among medical students. A replication of this study in a Swedish medical school confirmed these findings and also provided more direct evidence that the frustrated occupational ambitions of the father are visited upon the first-born son.

The question has been raised about how these various forms of status inconsistency are related to integration-disintegration. If we include in the definition of inconsistency, (1) status incongruence within the individual, (2) status discrepancy between husband and wife, and (3) status mobility as measured by a status difference between father and son, then I think we can infer with some assurance that status inconsistency will usually be a part of disintegration. Any change that affects status, e.g., technological changes, large cultural changes, changes in income, changes in education, changes in the power structure, or mobility and migration will almost certainly alter status unevenly so that inconsistency is increased.

It all argues, you see, for not taking social class or disintegration as global and undifferentiated concepts.

A third area of theory relates back to some of the metatheoretical points. I often have the feeling that your dependent variables don't seem very relevant to your independent variables. When I look at status and all the dependent mental health variables one might think of studying, I think of ones that seem a lot more relevant than your measures of psychiatric illness. I think for example, that things that I know nothing about, like clinical depression, sound more relevant to status differences in society (who wouldn't be depressed at being at the very bottom of the ladder?) Having an ulcer seems less relevant. Now, it often happens that what seems more relevant to us doesn't turn out to be more correlated. I'm quite aware of that, and that poses some interesting questions. But the whole problem of getting relevant dimensions and measures is one I think you were studying.

Freydberg: In essence, you're saying, it's more of a specificity you want here, a particular kind of status that give you this type of behavior, behavioral response, or dependent variable?

French: I think we'll put it this way: I think we ought to be more specific on our independent variable, whether it's status, or disintegration; I think we ought to be more specific on our dependent variables. There ought to be a large set of very specific ones.

I think we ought to be more specific in our hypotheses linking these independent and dependent variables. And these hypotheses really ought to be themes as illustrated in Figure 3; that is, sets of inter-linked hypotheses that say: "this specific aspect of the objective environment affects this aspect of the subjective or psychological environment, which produces this kind of response, conditioned by this kind of personality variable, which, in turn, produces this specific kind of mental health problem. So it's a theme involving a set of hypotheses, and all along the way I'm for being more analytical and less global in the concepts used.

Now, I must say that I picked this argument up from reading your proposal, I'm well aware of that. This is presented in your proposal, and so, if I'm not carrying coals to Newcastle, I'm saying, "well, go a bit further on that"; and also saying, "I had a hard time, when I read both the proposal and the notes of your Seminars, in seeing the specific theory."

I don't know anything about psychosomatic disease and that whole area, but I'm strongly in favor of the specificity hypothesis there. I think you ought to have the kinds of theories that would explain the fact that some people get ulcers, others get rheumatoid arthritis, and still others have asthma. This really goes back to metatheoretical conceptions: first, that everything is caused, and so there's some cause, some reason for differences; second, that we are at a stage now where we are able to discover these specific causes.

I would again adhere very strongly to a strategy of successive approximations in research. I know that Kurt Lewin was a great proponent of this and so is Alex Leighton, and I don't think there is any disagreement there. I think I'm saying now, I am more optimistic about your findings than you seem to be, in terms of where you are. So I would be ready for more specific hypotheses; at least I'd like to push in that direction.

There is one more theoretical point worth emphasizing. I mentioned personality variables, and to some extent some of the interest I have in self-identity theory, but now I would like specifically to talk about conditioning variables. These aren't completely and generally understood in all social science, and I don't think I have in any one place written enough about this, so let me take five minutes on this point.

I think I'd like to illustrate this with cross-cultural research. I have been involved, among other things, in doing cross-cultural studies, where I developed a point of view involving conditioning variables.

We got some findings in my early studies on the effects of participation (the effects of participation mainly in industrial situations) on several dependent variables; on satisfaction; on interpersonal relations within the group or organization; on productivity. Then the question arose, "Well, would these give you the same effects in an authoritarian culture, or other different cultures?"

These are the kinds of questions that the anthropologists have raised so consistently and so fruitfully that even the psychologists who really know nothing about anthropology are beginning to get infected with this bug and have started thinking about it. Then I replicated this study in Norway. All right, now, what might you get?

Well, you might get a replication in the sense that when you did the same thing over again you get the same result. We could say, "Well, now we can generalize a little more broadly to a larger sample." This doesn't say a thing about whether we could generalize to Sweden, or to Denmark, certainly not to China.

So, that raises still the question: Under what conditions does this hold? I simply know that it holds in places 1 and 2, and I don't know the conditions that make that the case. I haven't really gone very far replicating in every culture in the world.

But suppose we find cultural differences. When you find differences, then what do you do with them? With regard to this specific hypothesis about the effects of participation on production in a work group do we say, "We give it all up, there are no general laws?" No of course we don't say that. We say, "There must be something in the *conditions* that accounts for this difference."

I would like to propose that the way we ought to formulate that is not in terms of dichotomous difference such as the difference between men and women, but that you ought to conceptualize the difference, in this case between Norway and the United States, in terms of a variable rather than an all or none condition, and this conditioning variable, then should be stated in a three-variable hypothesis that can be tested in an analysis of variance by the interaction terms.

One can formulate the hypothesis abstractly: to the extent that variable C is present, A will cause B. In the absence of C, A will not cause B. That's the most abstract statement. In my studies, I was asking "What might be the difference between how participation might operate in this country and in Norway?" We thought that the legitimacy of participation seemed to be a relevant variable, a conditioning variable; that if people (and now this could be the society, the total culture, the factory, the work group) consider it legitimate that workers ought to participate in making certain kinds of decisions, and illegitimate if they're not permitted to participate in making these kinds of decisions, then according to this legitimacy of particpation, we should get either favorable or unfavorable effects on production and attitudes. If it's considered illegitimate, this participation should have unfavorable effects. Our findings tended to support this. With such an hypothesis I can generalize much more broadly, I can generalize about any culture you can name provided I can get a measure of the legitimacy or illegitimacy of participation. I can also talk about the differences between any factories within a culture. So I'm suggesting that we need to think about cultural differences, differences between organizations, differences between sexes, these kinds of categorical differences that we tend to start with, in terms of variables. That's where we should be headed, and we should try to think of these as having possible interaction effects.

I started out with personality. Let me come back to that and say that one of the most important conditioners, or set of conditioning variables, will be personality variables. The general principle here (and this is a simple extension of field theory as expounded by Gestalt psychology, by Kurt Lewin, and by lots of other people) is that behavior, including mental health and illness, is determined by the interaction of person and environment. If we want to study the effects of the environment—my interest and yours—we are still eventually going to have to take account of personality differences.

One man's meat is another man's poison, and we have to look at that. We then get the best understanding and the strongest correlation between environmental variables, on the one hand, and mental health variables, on the other, if we look at how they interact with conditioning personality variables.

So, if we're interested in role conflict, in an organization and its effect on mental health, we find over and over again, we get much higher relationships when we say: "Now that will vary depending upon whether a man is a rigid or a flexible personality." So we use the California Personality Inventory as a measure of flexibility-rigidity [8].

[8] Kahn, R. L., Wolfe, D. M., Quinn, R. P., Snoek, J. D., & Rosenthal, R. A. *Organizational stress: Studies in role conflect and ambiguity.* New York: John Wiley & Sons, 1964.

Sure enough, those who are rigid behave one way, those who are flexible behave in just the opposite way; that is, role conflict has an opposite effect on them. If you had not taken into account this conditioning variable and instead had lumped together the rigid and flexible people, the two would have cancelled out. You'd come to the wrong conclusion, that role conflict isn't affecting your dependent variable.

This has happened so frequently in our studies that we're again trying to pass a law about this, and say, "We don't want, in our program, ever to do a study without taking into account the conditioning, personality variables."

What are the relevant conditioning personality variables with respect to status in our society? Let me recommend some that we think are so powerful, important, and fruitful that other people ought to be studying them too, and that they ought to be considered in this program. One is achievement motivation. I see you've been reading about the achieving society here, and I'm sure most of you know more about McClellan's work and Atkinson's work than I do. But nevertheless, I keep getting this rubbed off on me from Jack Atkinson, who is, by the way, now a colleague of mine. I'm very convinced that his new developments, in which he distinguishes or breaks down achievement motivation into the motive to achieve success, and a separate motive to avoid failure, have real theoretical power. This has made me feel, in all the projects I'm doing, that there's a need to make this distinction.

We talk a lot about status striving. Another relevant kind of personality variable is the need for status. I think there is some such need inside the person. We have to look at his reaction to the status structure of society in terms of this need. Now, that also gets very close to the need for subjective public esteem; I think they might be identical.

My term subjective public esteem means: how the person thinks he is evaluated by some relevant public, that is, some reference group or reference figure. How much does your father respect and evaluate you, or your boss, or your group of professional colleagues in the world, or whatever your reference groups might be?

So there's a real question: Is there a basic, human need, similar to need achievement, to be valued by others in your reference groups? That gets awfully close, finally, to a need for self-esteem.

Frankly, I'm worried about these very closely overlapping needs, and I keep thinking about them and trying to make distinctions and so on. However, we have had more success in measuring the *level* of self-esteem as a personality variable. I've also found that the effect of the environment is entirely different, depending on whether the person is high in self-esteem or low [9]. So I have to treat self-esteem as an important conditioning variable.

I think that's enough on theory. Let me indicate the kinds of methodological issues somewhat more briefly, because they begin to stem from these theoretical issues. If you have an approach in which you are, let's say, more emphasizing analytical subparts, and subvariables, then I suggest you should measure all these, and it's a question of what intervening variables should you be looking for? How should you measure them? These are the kinds of questions we should ask. I think that I've already indicated that the conception of conditioning variables would lead me to think about relevant personality variables even in studies that focus primarily on the effects of the environment.

I think the kind of over-all strategy employed would lead to a lot of questions that come into design and sampling. When I read over your notes about whether you should select tracts or blocks, or do a random sampling of individuals, my strategy would be, as Kurt Lewin used to say, "Start strong." By that he meant (this is part of his strategy of

[9] Kay, E., Meyer, H. H., & French, J. R. P., Jr. Effects of threat in a performance appraisal interview. *Journal of Applied Psychology*, 1965, *49* (5), Pp. 311-317.

successive approximation), let's start out with good big, strong differences; and I would add, especially on the independent variable. You already are going to have to get a wide range of mental health for your other purposes of validating your measures of mental illness. But for this other purpose of understanding the effects of status, or disintegration, let's get good, big, strong differences of integration-disintegration or of status. This would be the strategy.

Then, methodologically, that would mean to me that you don't select individuals, because you're talking about some sort of a social system (I take it disintegration is a property of a social system or a social subsystem) that would be the thing you should start strong on, on status as a property of social systems. This leads to these suggestions: Instead of considering mainly blocks and census tracts, why don't we sample face-to-face groups, think about networks; select social organizations; think, within the work situation, about the face-to-face group? Why don't we sample families as the systems?

Well, I think I have thrown out far too many ideas, and I have even a larger number in my notes. Why don't we stop at this point and hear your ideas about where we'd like to pick up one of these? There's obviously a lot of interconnection, and I think by picking up one end of the handkerchief we'll eventually get to all four corners.

In conclusion, we have covered thirteen types of disintegration, presented four attempts at a refined definition of the integration-disintegration hypothesis, and closed with a challenging critique by John R. P. French.

7

Urban Residential Indicators of Integration-Disintegration

BERTON H. KAPLAN, Ph.D.

Seminar Participants

Isidor Chein, Ph.D.   Raymond Illsley, Ph.D.
Nicholas Freydberg, Ph.D.   Alexander Leighton, M.D.
John S. Harding, Ph.D.   Dorothea C. Leighton, M.D.
Lawrence Hinkle, M.D.   Jane M. Murphy, Ph.D.
Laurel Hodgden, Ph.D.   William F. Whyte, Ph.D.

INTRODUCTION *

As a demonstration of the variety of information that one can get on a residential classification basis concerning properties of populations living in any designated area, Dr. Isidor Chein enumerated a number of indices he has constructed by this means for New York City. These are available by census tracts in most instances, and even by blocks (from census tapes) if the expense of special tabulation is warranted. Through statistical procedures it is possible to depart from the tracts when the combining of contiguous areas becomes desirable. Among his indices is

* Written by Nicholas Freydberg, Ph.D.

one indicative of family disorganization, which includes such variables as proportion of married women not living with their husbands, etc. Another index deals with "socio-economic squalor," and refers to variables like proportion of families with incomes under $2,000, men in low occupations, unemployed, adults with less than high school education, etc. A third relates to socio-economic contrasts and consists of many of the variables in "socio-economic squalor" and is concerned with the variability (range) of these measurements within a tract. The belief is that this has relevance for cultural conflict and awareness of deprivation, since in areas where the range is great, there are likely to be tenement occupants close by the luxurious apartment houses and homes of the well-to-do. Then there are indices for the proportion of juveniles to total population, for population composition, household composition, status discrepancy (proportion of bread-winners whose incomes are above, equal to, or below their education level), and one defined as the functionless drop-out population, youths who are above a specified education level but are neither at school nor at work.

Dependent variables also are available information in New York City. Out-of-wedlock births, school drop-outs, 16-year-olds in continuation school, juvenile syphilis, truancy, and delinquency (based on Court appearance on a charge) are of relevance to Dr. Chein's project. As he views it, these represent violations of society's norms and reflect conditions that may lead people not to take these norms seriously. Indices like family disorganization, socio-economic squalor, socio-economic contrasts, juvenile and minority group density, etc., are built into a regression analysis schema in order to determine their separate impacts on the dependent variables.

The possible relationship of these indices and a cultural atmosphere that bears on the acceptance or rejection of the general social norms is certainly of interest to research as proposed in the present project, which is itself concerned with the impact of social disintegration on mental disorder. Among the advantages of this residential allocation of phenomena is the ability to locate deviant behavior in the areas where likelihood of it is great and where it is much less so. This is of value for the investigation of dynamics and process, as they are likely to be different where the deviant is moving with the predominant forces than where he is moving against them. Another analytic opportunity may be provided by discrepancies based on expectations of deviancy in each of these tracts (using the indices for predictions) and the actual incidence of this behavior.

A few questions were raised at this point. Conceding the wide prevalence of mental illness in these depressed areas of New York City, how do you link these areas to the city's social processes? One view expressed was that it was enough to get at what is linking the individual to the disease process. Relating the social processes of the city to the emergence of certain effects in the depressed areas would be carrying the question of dynamics back still farther and in the opposite direction. Then, how do you get beyond correlations and reach an understanding of causal relationships involved in these high rate tracts? The requirement for that may be some theory or theories of mental illness that define what the inquiry is about. Obtaining information of relevance to these theories is a function of the methodology.

The Family as a Social Process

A number of factors appeared to coalesce when the family came under inspection as the possible unit for the study of social process. For one thing, it could be a linking unit employable both in Nova Scotia and in an urban area. Further, the family measures shown to be available in the Chein presentation parallel many of those related to social disorganization in the earlier research. The family qualifies as a unit that can vary on a set of dimensions that are identifiable by research methods. As one participant pointed out, the meaning to children in Scarsdale of having several fathers is quite different as regards their mental health than the meaning it has to children in Puerto Rican Harlem.

Determining why some people become ill in well-integrated communities and others stay well in disintegrated ones may be feasible through the family context. One difficulty with the work place as a focus was that many other factors in the individual's life space could neutralize its effects, but the family is less subject to this possibility. All in all, the family unit is small enough for the observation of certain dynamic forces, and these are not so numerous or diffuse as to prevent the possibility of their observation over time. While the usual restrictions to generalization apply, the family unit has the advantage of being pervasive in Western culture, and the possibility exists of dynamic factors within the unit that may cut across prime areas of geography, population density, and even social barriers.

The proposal to focus on the family raised some issues. The question of whether you get high incidence of pathology in areas of high incidence of family disorganization is a different one than whether pathology is most likely to strike within the disorganized family. Both are implied in the summary of advantages listed above. If the family becomes the unit for observation as a social process in its own right, then what provision will be made for the measurement of the influence of social processes outside of the family that the family mediates to its members? One suggestion was to leave for the next step the interaction of the family with larger groups. Does exclusive concentration on the family neglect other systems that have relevance to mental health? Participation in religious and educational groups and in leisure activities is likely to be reflected somewhat in the family constellation, but does the family situation provide sufficient of the life situation of certain individuals and the different forces affecting them, such as the young and the old? Can the effect of the extent of overlap of the various interaction systems of the individual on his mental health be adequately assessed from the family focus? All foci have biases, the family focus excludes individuals who do not participate in family life.

The Nongeographic Approach

The nongeographic position was not buried by the agreement reached on the family unit. The contention here remains that, most likely, our society generates mental illness through inter-relations, and it is more to the question to tie into this by social units rather than geographic units. The complexity of an urban community, its many social groups and variety of on-going social processes, allows for the likelihood of mental illness to vary with the process and the group. A manageable and potentially more productive strategy may be to study one social process and one group at a time, rather than cutting across many of these as is probable by selecting residential areas.

The following discussion deals primarily with a presentation and critical examination of Isidor Chein's model of social disintegration, which is measured by socio-demographic indices.

EDITED TRANSCRIPT

Chein: I think I would like to draw a distinction in the light of the direction that the discussion is taking. In effect, the point was made that while we can start with any segment of the population, we can get all kinds of people in by moving to the relatives of the particular individuals that are taken. I doubt very much if the outcome would be a good one if one defined the population that way.

If you start, say, with a job population, and then move from there to a larger population, in terms of the people that are associated with the ones who are working in the job, I think we have practically nothing to go by as to the properties of the population that's being defined.

(Methodology (M)—population: If you are concerned about the definition of the population, you need to start with one you know something about. The definition of a population should be kept separate from the data collected about the population (as their families, etc.))

I can now make the distinction I referred to at the beginning. It seems to me if one wants to focus on any population, one can move out from that population for data of any kind about the population elements of the sample elements whether it's job data or anything else. But if one is concerned with the definition of a population, it seems to me one needs to define the population, to start with, as a population that one knows something about. So, if one starts with a job population, from this point of view, I think one is committed to taking the people on the job, or in the industry, or however it's structured, as the elements. About them we may find out all kinds of things about their families. If one starts with the residential population, one can find out about their jobs and whatever one can. But one should keep the definition of the population distinct from the data that one is collecting about the population.

(M—population: Selective factors operate in any given area: a job population eliminates unemployables; residential areas may have a socio-economic bias.)

I've already made the point that if one starts with a job population, there is a very marked bias with respect to the kinds of elements that would get into the population; this is perfectly all right if that's the population one wants to study. If one starts with the job population, one automatically eliminates the very young and the very old, the housewife, unemployables, and many others as elements of the population under study. There are also selective factors if one starts with any given area, but they are along different dimensions. They're in socio-economic dimensions, possibly in ethnic dimensions or what not.

(*M—population:* Unless job impact on mental health is the specific focus, the more strategic approach is a population defined in the community where there is census information.)

My own guess would be that in a study that isn't specifically focused on the impact of the job on the mental health of the workers, the more strategic approach is to go through a population defined in the community. Concerning such a population, there is a lot of information available, as of the census years, if one is in an area where there is a good deal of census information. I do have some notion of what's available in New York City and presumably in any other area of the United States since one could presumably get parallel information. I don't know if it would be desirable for me to run through some of the kinds of information that one can get from the census. If it is, I can give some indication of the kinds of variables I'm working with.

Murphy: As you're doing this, could you tell us something about what you have in mind geographically in New York so that we could think of a particular area as you're talking?

(*M—population:* Chein project is working with all New York City divided into census tracts.)

Chein: Right now, I'm working with all of New York City divided into tracts. Most of these are census tracts. What I was looking for was information that would have some theoretical bearing on the generation of social climates that are hospitable to contranormative behaviors—that is, behaviors that violate the norms of society at large—and to the relative impotence of societal norms in regulating the behaviors of individuals. Note that I am speaking of the norms of the society as a whole, and not of the particular societal segment with which we happen to be dealing. Thus, some of the norms of a subsociety may themselves be *contranormative,* in the sense that I have given to the latter term.

(Forty-five variables have been classified into domains. One is indicative of family disorganization: proportion of married women not living with husbands, couples not living in own home, etc.)

All of the kinds of information that I'm going to mention were available for census tracts. I started out with some forty-five variables classified in domains and subdomains. I have to make these linguistic distinctions because of the nature of my operation. I also get into universes and subuniverses.

Let me just mention the domains, which are the simplest. The first one consists of a group of variables that are in some sense indicative of a *degree of family disorganization* that is prevalent in the area. For instance, one of our variables is the proportion of women who have been married but are not living with their husbands at the time of the census, and one can similarly get the proportion of men who have been married but are at the time of census not living with their wives. Another variable from the census is the proportion of the population that is not living with a relative, and another is the proportion of married couples that are not living in their own homes. I've also included in this group the proportion of women in the labor force. It is debatable whether it belongs in this group, but for various reasons I preferred to see it there.

(*M—population:* Another set of variables deal with "socio-economic squalor"; proportion of families with income under $2,000; men in low occupations; unemployed; less than high-school education; overcrowded homes.)

A second set of variables has to do with what I called "socio-economic squalor." Here we have a variety of variables that have to do with the question of families with incomes under some specified amount (we were working with $2,000 as the specified amount), the proportion of unemployed men, the proportion of people with less than some specified amount of education (below high school level), the proportion of men in the labor force who are in low occupations, unskilled labor.

Among the socio-economic squalor variables, we have the percentage of homes that are overcrowded. We've been working with the old census criterion of more than 1½ persons per room. In the 1960 census, the main tabulation that the census made was one person per room (the standards have gone up). But, for New York City at least, there is available the 1½ person criterion, and this is also tabulated by the census but not published on a census tract bases, which means it's relatively easy to get from the census if they continue to do this in the future.

(*M—population:* A third set deals with socio-economic contrasts. Most variables in "squalor" are bases for variability measures. Where greater variability exists within a tract and with adjoining ones, greater cultural conflict is likely and deprivation more apparent.)

My third group of variables is a fairly complicated one: those concerned with socio-economic contrasts. Most of the variables that I mentioned under socio-economic squalor can become bases of variability measures, that is you can get some measure of income variability dealing with the inter-quartile range of income. Unfortunately, these relatively simple measures of socio-economic contrasts turn out to be quite defective, mainly as a consequence of the extremely skewed distributions. We were, however, able to derive a number of contrast measures, for instance, by comparing each tract with the tracts adjacent to it.

In theoretical terms, my interest in the variability measures stems from the notion that the more variable, i.e., in socio-economic terms, a given area is, (a) the greater the cultural conflict possibilities via the several social classes that are present, and (b) the relative deprivation of individuals at the low end becomes sharply focused—you've got the evidence right in front of your eyes.

A. Leighton: May I ask what is size of the population in the tract?

Chein: Cenus tracts vary, both in population size and area, from a handful of people in a large area (Central Park, for instance, constitutes two census tracts, populated presumably by the caretakers and their families) to thousands of people crowded into a few square city blocks. To protect the privacy of the residents, the census does not provide separate data on the virtually unpopulated tracts so that these cannot be utilized. Even so, there are many census tracts without large enough resident populations for reliable indices so that, in many instances, we combined adjacent tracts (on the basis of similarity of profiles across our thirty-three basic indices, length of common border, etc.). Thus, for 1950, we had 1,371 tracts (i.e., census tracts or combinations thereof) and, for 1960, 1,427 tracts. These tracts are not as variable in population size as the original census tracts and account for virtually the total population of New York City—let us say, then from about 4,500 to about 7,000 persons per tract in most cases.

(M—population: The fourth set deals with juvenile population: the ratio of 16-19-year-old boys to adults, and for various combinations of age levels and sex.)

Now, for my fourth group of variables, I was interested in population composition on the basis of age and sex.

For example, one of the variables I'm working with is the ratio of 16-19-year-old boys to the adult population, and I've got this for various combinations of age-by-sex. Another kind of measure would be the relative number of various age-sex groups per block. One can do this per acre if you have the acreage of the census tracts, which wasn't available when I started but which, at least in New York City, is now available on the 1960 basis.

Harding: Could you state again the common theme of these indices?

(*M—population:* The fifth group is concerned with population composition and involves Negro, Puerto Rican, and white classification.)

Chein: The fourth group is juvenile population composition. My fifth group is also concerned with population composition and involves the Negro-Puerto Rican-white classification, and a variety of indices that can be developed out of this. For various strategic reasons, for instance, I found it useful to count as follows: the proportion of the non-Puerto Rican population that is Negro, the proportion of the non-Negro population that is Puerto Rican, and the proportion of the total population that is Negro or Puerto Rican. I've also got a foreign-born in there as a variable.

Whyte: Including Puerto Rican?

(*M—population:* All these variables except a few in the third group, are available from census publications or tapes.)

Chein: No, this is non-Negro, non-Puerto Rican foreign-born. All of these, with the exception of some of the variables in my third group are quite easily obtainable from census publications, or are available on tapes.

There was a variable I was very much interested in, which for certain reasons I knew was quite misleading in New York City. This had to do with population mobility in terms of my central interests. It was very easy to pick up from the census the proportion of the population which, at the time of the cenus, was not living at the same address as they had been the preceding year, or not living in the same county as they had been in the preceding year. I once used this variable and called it "new faces."

But there is a good deal of evidence that in New York City, these new-faces variables mean quite different things in the different boroughs. In Manhattan, for instance, it's largely made up of the better-off individuals who have moved back to the city after their children have grown up. In the Bronx, it's the out-pouring from the Manhattan slum areas and so it becomes a quite confused variable for my purposes. I realized what I really wanted was a tabulation of this based on the youth. Once I started thinking in terms of special tabulations I just let myself go, because if you're going to do one you might as well do another one, and pretty soon, depending on how you count them, you've got some 600 special tabulations coming from the Census Bureau.

The significance of this is: Once we have paid for the programming, it becomes much more economical to get this kind of tabulation for any place. We sort of expect that it would be, so let me give you some notion of what these special tabs are. I have no doubt but that other people can invent others, because all you have to do is look at what the census asks for, and then you can figure out how you would like to have it broken up.

(M—population: Special census tabulations have given us household composition broken down in many ways; e.g., for average 16-19-year-old boys, number of children and adults in his household.)

We have a group of variables related to the family composition broken down in various ways. To give a typical example, we will have for 1960 (this is no longer possible for 1950) for the average 16-19-year-old Negro boy how many adults are in his family and how many children are in his family, that is, the proportion of children to adults in his family. We can get a similar index for the average 16-19-year-old girl, and we can get it for other age levels.

Murphy: Does this mean family in the extended sense, or the household?

Chein: The household. It's probably misleading to talk about any of this in terms of family household systems that are involved in the census statistics, although it's also possible to derive families. We haven't asked for this. The indices we're talking about now are merely household indices, but it is obvious that you can derive families from one indice that I mentioned before: married couples not living in their own household. This means that they're living in somebody else's household, and so the immediate family can be distinguished in the sense that it's there in the census. In 1960, and undoubtedly for all future censuses, this will be unchanged, which makes it a lot easier to get at.

(*M—population:* Another of our variables is status discrepancy, the proportion of main breadwinners whose incomes are above or below, or deviant with regard to their educational level.)

Another kind of variable has to do with status discrepancy. What we actually have done is a total cross-tab of income by education. We then set our plotting points as to what discrepancy between income and education we will regard as deviant. Once we do that, we can then get counts of the number of, or, say, the proportion of youth in the various age-by-sex strata living in households where the income of the main breadwinner is above his educational level, or below, or simply deviant with regard to his educational level.

(*M—population:* The same things are being done for occupational level, but the information from the census interviews is not as reliable.)

Each of these, theoretically, has a different kind of significance. We're having the same cross-tab made by occupational level. This is one that I don't trust as much because I think this is probably the most fallible one of the census indices, where they classify people in terms of occupational level. It's fallible, not because of what happens after the census interviews are conducted, but because of the census interviews, the kind of thing that's available for classification is of a dubious character.

(M—population: We have obtained a land-use map from the City Planning Commission which makes possible a variety of indices of the distance every tract is from various kinds of areas: industrial, business, small residences, tenements, large apartment houses, etc.)

Then, for New York City (this is now no longer in the census) we were able to get from the City Planning Commission a land-use map of New York City that makes it possible to develop a whole variety of indices based on the distance of any given census tract from an area of industrial concentration, or from an area of business concentration, or from an area of essentially small residential houses, as against large apartment houses and tenements.

We got involved in this because although I was interested in the kinds of hypotheses associated with the Chicago Ecological School, New York City isn't laid out in concentric circles. But the basic issues are issues that don't have to do with concentric circles, they have to do with distances from specified kinds of areas.

Harding: Do you take into account lines of transportation at all, such as the subway?

(M—population: We have yet to develop a way to take account of transportation lines. Evidence exists that narcotics use tends to move along subway lines.)

Chein: I haven't figured out a good way to do this yet. I would very much like to. The trouble here is not with the subways, those are relatively easy. It's the bus lines that drive me mad. I would very much hope to be able to develop some kind of index on this basis. For instance, in the drug addiction studies, there was some indication that spread tends to move along the subway lines. You have an area of high narcotics use and another area that is low; if they're connected by subway lines, there's a greater likelihood that the second area will get some narcotics use, compared to an area not on a direct subway line. But this is just a rough impression. I haven't worked this out systematically, but it's a fairly obvious one which would seem to be of some significance. This gives you some idea of the variety of information that one can get on a residential classification basis concerning the properties of populations living in any designated area. *Murphy:* Have you carried the analysis far enough that you can say which of your five or six factors are found together in particular areas, such as family disorganization and so forth?

(M—population: Census tracts when deficient in population were combined by comparing profiles with adjacent tracts, based on thirty-three indices, which provided correlations involving both shape and level of similarity.)

Chein: I can tell you something about this because it was our basis for combining census tracts when a population was deficient in a given tract. We took the thirty-three indices that we already had available and started with the deficient tracts. We computed an intraclass correlation across the profile between every one of these tracts and every tract adjacent to it. This was our major criterion for combining: they should be similar in profile. The intraclass correlation involves not only the shape of the profile but also the level achieved, and so it's an ideal kind of measure of profile similarity.

There were other criteria, such as the length of the common boundary. Where we combined two tracts, if the population was still deficient, then we again looked at all of the adjacent tracts.

(M—population: Age composition varies by tracts. Some have lots of young children and few teen-agers. Sex ratios vary enormously.)

It's also really remarkable how the age composition varies. There are tracts where you will find hardly any young children. There are tracts where you will find lots of young children, but you won't find teen-agers. You'll find them, but the ratios vary enormously. There's considerable variation in sex ratios from tract to tract. These are things that one doesn't ordinarily expect to get much variation in. There are reasons for this, areas of new settlement, completely new buildings where young married people tend to move and as a result, there are no teen-agers there.

(M—population: Dependent variables are available information in New York City, such as: out-of-wedlock births, school drop outs, 16-year-olds in continuation schools, juvenile syphilis, 10th grade truancy.)

I should have mentioned that, at least for New York City, dependent variables become available information. Thus, we are working with delinquency. There are also out-of-wedlock childbirths. We are also working with an index of school dropouts: the number of boys and girls who elect to leave school. They must go into the continuation schools for a year (they can't just elect to leave school at 16; they are supposed to be working to be allowed to leave school before they are 17 years old). It provides a convenient counting point. All one has to do is to go to the continuation schools, collect the thousands of roll books, and locate the individuals who are listed there in their census tract. At any rate we've done this for 1950 and for 1960 so that this is available.

I mentioned out-of-wedlock childbirths, juvenile syphilis is another one. This is not at age 16; we've extended our age here, actually I think we include through 21 as the base figure. This is the easiest one to get because the Department of Health has them on IBM cards; all we have to do is census tract them, then we can make our tabulations. I picked on syphilis rather than venereal disease in general, which is also available, because the figures on syphilis are probably much more trustworthy. If a doctor doesn't report it, but turns it into a lab, you get the lab report; eventually it gets to the Board of Health. With gonorrhea, if the doctor decides to do his own lab test as many do, which they will rarely do for syphilis, you get that complete sector suppressed, so syphilis seemed much better. All that you're losing are the cases where the doctor makes a clinical diagnosis and doesn't bother with the lab test and doesn't report either. You may even get those if the same case shows up at another doctor's office.

A. Leighton: How about the ones who don't go to a doctor at all? The primary stage of syphilis may be gone through without too much of a problem.

Chein: You don't get them.

A. Leighton: How big a problem do you think this is?

Chein: I could only guess, and it would be a totally uninformed guess. I would assume that a substantial number of individuals are undetected on that basis, and what's more that it would make for some systematic bias. I think it's less likely that the higher socio-economic strata of the population would go undetected than the lower ones. This is still a guess. If this guess is valid, it would tend to make some of the correlations we have obtained underestimates. Syphilis correlates .72 with family disorganization, .62 with socio-economic squalor, .29 with socio-economic contrasts, .45 with the composition of the juvenile population, and .63 with the minority group population density. Most of these correlations are substantially lower than the corresponding correlations with the other indices of contranormative behavior.

Freydberg: Do you have any other kind of dependent (contranormative) variables?

Chein: I had hoped to include truancy data, but this did not prove to be feasible. We do have component indices. Thus, the over-all delinquency index is actually a composite of nine measures.

Harding: What delinquency statistic or statistics do you use?

(M—population: The source of data for delinquency statistics is a court appearance on a charge. Charges also are classified and available by tract.)

Chein: Well, the actual index is a complicated one because it takes into account the stratification of the population by age and by sex, and four varieties of offenses by males in the 16-through 19-year old age range, but the source of the data is a court appearance on a charge. In effect, my reasoning was that this is better than a police blotter because it implies that there's at least enough evidence to bring the person to court, and also that it is better than final disposition, in part because final disposition is complicated by various laws that have to do with changing of charges and so forth. In addition, a certain amount of experience has indicated that the final disposition is more likely to be "not guilty" if the person has enough money to stick it out, to hire a lawyer, and to pay the lawyer to invest his time. I thought the least vulnerable point was the point of being brought up in court on charges.

We've also got the charges classified by tab which we plan to use in another analysis. The index takes into account a stratification of charges. We have four classes of charges, but we have much more detailed classifications summarized by tracts. We have them by census tract too, which we plan to use in another kind of an analysis of the data.

(M—population: Behaviors such as delinquency, school drop outs, etc., represent violations of society's norms. They reflect conditions that may lead people not to take these norms seriously.)

I shall try to explain what I'm getting at, or at least what I think I'm getting at with these groupings of variables. In effect, starting with the assumption that behavior such as delinquency, school drop outs, and so on, represent behaviors that violate the norms of the society, I was thinking in terms of a variety of conditions that might lead individuals not to take these norms seriously. I thought of each of these groups of variables as getting at a different kind of social factor that would lead to widespread disrespect for such norms. For example, the family taken as a major instrument of the transmission of norms: if there is a great deal of family disorganization, this might generate a condition in which there is a breakdown in the ability of families to fulfill this function. Socio-economic squalor might conceivably have this kind of effect in terms of "nothing is worthwhile." Nothing worse can happen to me than has happened. There is nothing to look forward to. One is essentially trapped, and so there's no premium in respecting any norms. Socio-economic contrasts are brought out in the culture-conflict sense. That is, as was indicated earlier, you've got two sets of norms. Taking any set of norms seriously becomes a more difficult task, and also in the sense of intensification of relative deprivation for the people at the low end of the scheme.

As for the juvenile population density, my reasoning was that where young people are richly available to support one another, the relative degree of adult control over the youth diminishes in a variety of ways. The minority group population density is relevant in terms of groups that tend to be the focus of all kinds of deprivations, and all of these factors tend to be at work here.

(M—population: Indices such as family disorganization, socio-economic squalor, socio-economic contrasts, juvenile and minority group density are built into a regression analysis scheme to study their interactions in order to determine their separate impact on the dependent variables.)

All of this is built into a complicated scheme of regression analysis, the purpose of which is to be able to study interactions among these variables in terms of the impact on the dependent variables, and also to give some differential weights to them. So far as knowledge of things like delinquency is concerned, we know enough by now, I think, to say that if you can think of something wrong with an environment, you'll find it in areas of high delinquency, but this raises the question: Are some of these badnesses there simply because they go along with other forms of badness, or are they actually playing a role in the incidence of contranormative behavior?

(*M—population:* The significance for this project is the possible relation between these social indices and a subcultural atmosphere that bears on acceptance or rejection of the general social norms.)

In order to resolve this, we have to be able to give some kind of rating to various factors. Fortunately, they don't vary perfectly, one with another, so that one can study the relative impact of various kinds. But for our own immediate purposes here, I think what is significant for us is the relation that I see between these various social indices, and a general cultural or subcultural atmosphere that has bearing on the acceptance or rejection of the general social norms.

There may be special norms within the subnorms, but there are also common norms that are shared by the entire society, such as the norms of law abidingness. Even in the most non-law abiding circles, there is an acknowledgment of the general society norms. It's not unusual, for instance, for a father who is himself a criminal to become quite abusive to his son who's following his footsteps because the son isn't behaving in a respectable fashion. That was the general scheme of things that dictated my selection of variables to work with. There are obviously other ways of thinking, but they could lead to very similar selections; obviously there's overlap between my selections and some of those that you have used in the past for quite different reasons.

(*M—population:* To begin with, deviant behavior has different meanings where it is common from where it is not. Two other factors are of interest: (1) the expected incidence of each form of deviant behavior, based on these social variables, and (2) the actual incidence level.)

There's one other aspect of what I'm doing which may have some relevance. It starts with the notion that deviant behavior must have different meanings in contexts in which deviancy is common, than in a context in which deviancy is not common. Now, with the scheme of analysis that I'm using for every one of the tracts in the city, I come up eventually with two major factors. One is the expected degree of incidence, based on all these social variables, of each of the forms of deviant behavior that is embodied in my dependent variables. Maybe you're not going to think of syphilis as a form of deviant behavior, but it involves, among other things, not doing the things that would prevent syphilis, as well as that it is contracted from certain forms of contact. The same is true of out-of-wedlock childbirths. It isn't only the fact that out-of-wedlock relations are involved, but also the fact that precautions aren't taken reflects a kind of deviant behavior.

(*M—population:* This makes possible a classification of tracts according to whether expectation is low, medium, or high, and according to whether incidence is above, below, or equal to expectation. In some way, tracts that have more than is expected are different from those that have less or equal expectation.)

We also have an actual incidence level, which makes it possible to classify tracts into sets or blocks according to whether the expectation is low, medium, or high, and according to whether the actual incidence is above, below, or equal to the expectation. This defines, in effect, nine sets of tracts for each of which some kind of different pattern exists. In some way, the tracts that have more than is expected on the basis of general trends are different from those that have less and these are different from those that are conforming tracts. This defines for me, at least, residential sections within which individuals live who behave in some deviant fashion, so one can classify individuals according to this kind of schema of social settings. If you put together the classifications for a variety of indices of deviant behavior, it becomes more than nine sets of tracts. I'm interested in the sets of tracts for a variety of special analytical reasons, but I think that they offer an interesting base from which to examine social data concerning deviant behavior in general. They also offer the possibility of investigating some interesting hypotheses. For instance, the hypothesis that formally similar contranormative behaviors carried out by persons in different kinds of tracts are socio-dynamically and psychodynamically different. Or that the different modal contranormative behaviors in different kinds of tracts are psychodynamically alike.

Now, I can't possibly get this analysis completed in time for this to make a difference in the planning of the study, but if the study is done in New York City, and on a regional basis, then by the time the study is in its last phases, it will be possible to say at least what kind of areas these were within the framework of this schema.

Hinkle: I'd like to comment on that if I may because I think the aim, or the problem, comes down to what question the study is going to ask. The census tract is a geographic area. You pointed out earlier that an employment group is a population, highly biased, selected by virtue of the fact that these people are at one place of employment, or in one type of employment.

Again, I think that we have to face the fact that within modern societies, especially large complex modern communities such as New York City, any sort of arbitrary area, such as a census tract, is nothing more than a traditional convenience, a sort of geographic unit in which to accumulate data.

It's very true that a great deal of valuable information is available on the basis of these things, and it's surely true that this is a manner in which one can ascertain the geographic prevalence and incidence of certain types of phenomena. But whether this is a good way of tying into social processes, to social organizations, is another thing entirely.

I thought, perhaps, of examining this from the point of view of a relatively small social organization we all know very well. The medical center here is a functional social grouping. If we look at the people who make up this population, we see that the unit has senior physicians, junior members, and the training staff, it has still other people who work in the higher technical categories, volunteers, technical assistants, nurses, and others who carry out porter and cleaning functions. Each of these groups work together in this particular social unit and in this geographical area. But in this great community of which they're a part, they live in widely separate areas, but not entirely random areas, either.

(M—population: Most likely, our society generates mental illness through interrelations as part of a social process. It is more to the question to tie into this by social units rather than geographic areas.)

The physicians in our hospital live in Pelham, they live across the bridge in Englewood. Some of them live up around Rye. Some of them live on the East Side of Manhattan and down along the Village, but they are not randomly distributed over New York City. In fact, the junior physicians live in a little enclave of special housing near the hospital and down in Stuyvesant Town. If you turn to the technical assistants, the nurses, the lab technicians, you'll find some of them live in the Bronx, and some of them live in Queens. The hospital volunteers, the ladies in pink, I find almost universally come from that area on the East Side that is somewhere between Fifth and near Park. The technical assistants, the cleaning people and so forth, are concentrated around areas of Harlem.

Now, here is a social organization in which the geographic elements are widely distributed. If we turn around, I suppose we'd go out to one of these places, such as Rye, where the doctors live, which incidentally is a part of New York, but it isn't part of New York City. It's a part of the social organization. If you look at the people there, you will find that living in this community are a group of other people with whom these professional people are interrelating, most of whom work in New York, but not randomly in New York: in Wall Street, in the Madison Avenue area, in certain of the large corporations that could be named almost for each community, in the UN.

There would be others in this professional group such as the doctors and lawyers to that immediate community. Also, within that community are retail trades people (service people who live and work in that community) and other service people, the police, domestic servants who wouldn't live in Rye or Pelham, or who would be more likely to live over in an area of Portchester.

Here is the way these things interrelate. If you cut across a census tract, that's like sampling a bee hive with a meat cleaver. It's an area of the city. Insofar as you pick up neighborhoods like Harlem, you have a certain homogeneity, but I think that the thing that you have to ask yourself is: How are you going to tie into this? Are you going to tie into it in terms of social process as an intercommunication, or are you going to tie into this in terms of geographic areas? In each case you're asking a different kind of question.

It seems to me most likely that our society generates in some way forms of mental illness. It generates it through the social interrelations and as part of the social process. We should sample social units and not geographic areas.

(*M—population:* Sampling on the basis of social process is good if the kind of sampling is related to the dependent variables. Occupational settings are not necessarily distributed the way mental illness is.)

Chein: I have two comments on this: one is that I agree with the thinking clearly, but not with the methodology. I think that sampling on the basis of social process would be good if one had some reason to believe that the kind of sampling going on is related to the dependent variables. As is, it's perfectly true that people who become mentally ill are in some kind of occupational setting. It's not necessarily true that these occupational settings are distributed the way mental illness is, and it's also not necessarily true that their experience in the occupational setting was the social process which was most responsible for the illness.

(*M—population:* The sampling is of individuals about whom you want to know the kinds of social settings and social processes in which they are enmeshed. The issue is how to select the elements that enable you to find these, not what are your independent variables.)

Now, it seems to me that the sampling, whether it's done in the occupational setting, or done in the residential setting, or done in some other fashion, is the sampling of individuals about whom one wants to know the kinds of social processes in which they are enmeshed. Now, if the focus was on the role of occupational setting in mental illness, those social processes would be most clearly known and most pursuable by taking your elements in common occupational settings, interrelated with one another, but not knowing that that is the key thing to study. It seems to me, one way or another, one wants elements where one is then to puruse the various kinds of social settings that they get involved in, and the kinds of social processes that they become subject to. The issue that's involved here is how do you select your elements, not what are your independent variables going to be.

There's one thing to be said about the census tract that hasn't been said so far: this is something that we know is very highly related to the distribution of all kinds of deviant behavior. In effect, knowing the properties of census tracts yields very high predictability of incidence, not of which particular individuals in these tracts will become deviant, but the sheer incidence of deviancy.

If you go back to Lander's study of delinquency in Baltimore, a multiple correlation of over .80 is nothing to be sneezed at, in terms of the distribution of this particular form of deviant behavior. In New York City, in Manhattan, I got a multiple "r" of about .80 with the incidence of drug involvement among the youth. In the Bronx, I got a multiple "r" separately of about .80. In Brooklyn, it was considerably lower, still about .60, and lower because you actually have a very much smaller range of drug involvement rates. So, in effect, we're dealing here with a set of variables that we know to be related to delinquency or drug addiction. You can start with Faris and Dunham on the distribution of mental illness, for these are things that we know, at least in the gross, are related. We have a basis for sampling elements in terms of contexts that are demonstrably relevant to the incidence of various forms of deviant behavior. Relevant to, of course, doesn't necessarily indicate the nature of the causal process. To start with, we know there is this relevance, and it's a very high degree of relevance.

(*M—population:* If commitment is in New York City, we are better off geographically because of rich resources. If smaller city where high percentage of workers are in a few industries and live nearby, it remains a question of emphasis.)

Whyte: If the decision is that the cases will be found in New York City, or the population to be studied be in that metropolitan area, then I think it pretty well follows from what has been said before that it's probably a better bet to start on a geographical basis than to start from employment, because in the plant individuals are scattered. On a geographical base, you'll go light on the organizational situation, but maybe you're better off in knowledge, especially having rich resources as Dr. Chein has.

I think that's very important background, but it still leaves unresolved the methodology regarding how you're going to figure out the dynamics. I think the argument could look different if we weren't committed to New York City as a base of operations. I think wherever you'd go, except in a very small community, the emphasis would have to be either in a geographical area, or on an organization, but it's possible to pick certain moderate-sized communities (Corning, as an example) where, if you started on people working in the Glass Works, a very high percentage of them will be living in Corning and immediate environs. If you start in the community, a very large percentage of those people will be working in the Corning Glass Works, in one or another part. There would still be the question of emphasis, where you're going to put your real, primary effort. But you'd be hedging your bets a bit, it seems to me. If you start with New York City (and there are many good reasons for doing so), I think the kind of materials that Dr. Chein is presenting and what he could develop on this are very powerful arguments, but I think certain things follow out of a choice of New York City that don't necessarily follow in the abstract. I think a decision is even open as to where the study is to be located.

(*M—population:* There are some advantages to doing the project in New York City in terms of professional and information sources. The grant does not limit us, New York or another urban area, or both are possible.)

A. Leighton: Let me make a comment on this point. There are a great many practical advantages to doing the project in New York City, in terms of New York medical sources being there, and it's much easier to do work out from that base than having all the problems we have in maintaining the one in Nova Scotia. Then, there are the advantages of New York, that we have both the work that has been mentioned today and that Hinkle and his workers have engaged in work with particular industries. But so far as the commitments of the Program are concerned, the terms of our grant do not limit us. In fact, it specifically states in the application that we might choose to work in New York, but we might choose to work somewhere else. We might work both of these if we had the resources.

I want to ask two interrelated questions that pertain to the one Dr. Hinkle raised, or maybe it's one of his questions in a somewhat different form. Taking off from the geographic area in the city and the geo-behavioral environment, there are two types of linkage that I would be very much interested in hearing some ideas expressed upon. One is how you would relate to this kind of condition. Take the worst areas for all of your indicators, the malfunction where you get a type of region that promotes deviancy as a social process. How do you link the processes of the city that produce these kinds of areas, or is this considered an irrelevant question and you simply take the areas as given? Or is it possible to think of the study as being concerned with how the city functions to produce such areas, and how these, in turn, affect mental health?

(*Social process:* The likelihood of wide prevalence of mental illness in these depressed areas is great. But how do you link these areas to the city's social processes? And, how do you get beyond correlation and understand causal relationships in the prevalence of mental illness in these areas?

Question two. If we start with the conception of facts deduced from either incidence or prevalence studies in these depressed areas of maximum deviancy, we're going to come up with a very wide prevalence of psychiatric disorders. I think this is a very safe bet because of the work that has already been done. They show low correlated SES levels; there's a correlation between general physical ill health and psychiatric disorders, and there's a correlation between various types of deviant behavior, such as drug use and alcoholism, and other forms of psychiatric disorder. All the arrows point in the direction of very high correlation if you were working in one of these areas. But how do you go from correlation to an understanding of the cause and effect relationship? Where you're working with youth, with drug users who are born into it, it seems to me you don't have these questions of which is cart and which is horse nearly as strongly as you do when you're concerned with the mental health of people who are a good deal older, many of whom have moved into the area, or the boy whose parents moved into the area because, in one way or another, they couldn't cope with the less deviant type of environment.

I'm really raising two questions: How do you link these depressed areas to the social processes of the city as a whole, and, on the other hand, how do you get beyond correlation and understand causal relationships that are involved in the high prevalence of mental illness in such an environment?

(*Social process:* Linking the social processes of the city to the emergence of depressed areas is carrying the question of dynamics a step farther. It's enough to get at what is linking the individual to the disease process. As to the causal process, you've got to work with some theory that defines what we're inquiring about. How you get relevant information is a question of methodology.)

Chein: It seems to me that the question of how you link the social processes of the city to the emergence of such areas is carrying the question of the dynamics a step further. It's going in the other direction.

Murphy: Dynamics of the individual or the social system?

Chein: Well, in the total causal process, if "a" is causing "b," but "c" is causing "a," and "d" is causing "c," and you keep going forever, eventually you'll get to "c," again, causing something else. Now, it seems to me that it's enough of a bite to get at what is linking the individual to the disease process, to the deviant behavior at one level, without asking how that has come about. But on the second question, of peering at the causal process, it seems to me you can ask the same questions that you have asked in any setting. You have got to work with some theory or some set of theories that define the thing that we are inquiring about. The question of where you get relevant information, whether you get it by asking people, or you try to get it in some other fashion, is a question of methodology. Suppose you take your industrial setting as your sampling case, it doesn't necessarily follow that, insofar as your getting interview information, the best place to interview the person is in the factory. It may well be that the best place to interview him is at home without his knowing that you know that he works in this factory. But those are questions of method, not of the basic strategy of your study. But no matter what context I got the person in, I would still be concerned with the questions of what are the stresses and strains to which those who fall by the wayside are subject, and which others are, either in some way able to overcome or don't experience these.

(*Social process:* The issue under discussion is not what you study, but how do you indicate the individuals to be studied. These should be defined separately.)

The issue we've been discussing is not the issue of what you study. The issue we've been discussing is how do you indicate the individuals to be studied? We haven't talked about how do you decide that they're mentally ill or not mentally ill. We haven't talked much about the strategic lines of investigation to try to learn what has been acting on the individual. We touched on this in earlier sessions, but those are questions of what to study, not whom to study, and it seems to me that what to study is defined independently of the whom to study.

The next two chapters (Chapters 8 and 9) consist of summaries of the presentations on the family made to the Seminar by Harold Feldman, Ph.D., and Mirra Komarovsky, Ph.D. The summary of Seminar ideas on how to study family processes and mental illness are included now as an introduction to these two chapters. Also, especially, see Isidor Chein's list of dimensions of family solidarity at the end of this summary.

Summary [1]

Seminar 6 concerned itself with the family's role in the proposed research, dealing with the pros and cons for employing it as an independent or intervening variable, or as the dependent variable. In addition, the discussion covered a number of dimensions of family life possibly related to the mental health of its members, the availability of these dimensions to measurement, and relevant research concerned with any of these factors.

THE FAMILY AS THE DEPENDENT OR INDEPENDENT VARIABLE

Arguments favoring the family as the dependent variable net down to these points. If interest lies in the causal implications of various patterns of family life, it is necessary to pick up the psychiatric reaction in any member. This would seem indicated for the collection of appropriate data on the interdependence of family members, as, for example, resistance to therapeutic intervention for an ill member, or transfer of symptoms in the event of another's recovery. The child, so often the focus of interest, is not only affected, he is in his own right an affector. In this regard, there are discrepancies in the perception of events among family members, indicating a need for reliance on more than one source in the family. One instance cited was where husbands and wives differed significantly on the amount of time each estimated that they spent talking to each other.

Evidence mounts on the considerable influence of the family on the

[1] Prepared by Nicholas Freydberg, Ph.D.

mental health of its members. A study of 850 Syracuse couples shows a curvilinear relationship in marital satisfaction over time that closely parallels data on proneness to psychiatric disorder found in the Midtown Manhattan Survey and other research. As people move from the honeymoon period (early 20's) to the 40's and 50's, marital satisfaction drops, and psychiatric disorder goes up. Later marital satisfaction rises and proneness to disorder goes down. A powerful indicator of psychic stress in the Midtown project was family worries. An index of perception of family cohesiveness distinguished, almost without overlap, between juvenile drug users and non-drug users, even when controlling for race and delinquency.

Social agencies have found it most productive to deal with the multiproblem family as a unit, and a number of psychiatric clinics likewise are, whenever possible, including the family of the psychiatric patient in the therapeutic relationship. The family crisis research of Caplan and Rapoport concentrates on this unit, and this is the direction of Spiegel and Kluckhohn who take as their focus divergent cultural values between the family and the community, and the consequent role conflict in the family, with effects for each member's psychodynamics.

The proponents of the use of the family as an independent or intervening variable, rather than the dependent variable, contend that in the latter event single individuals would be ruled out. The result would be to ignore certain factors related to mental health as this segment has a higher probability rate for mental illness. Then, if the influence of other aspects of the environment, such as the work-place, are to be considered in addition to the family, this is a feasible procedure only through individuals.

A commitment to investigate the validity of assessing an individual's mental health by survey methods, with the family as part of his environment, already exists, additional research in connection with it is in progress, and this focus cannot be abandoned. Related is the method of classification of individuals on a mental health continuum ranging from A to D. Families cannot be classified in this manner or in any comparable way; dealing with them as the dependent variable would require an entirely different rating design. If the research is directed at effects on the individual, in terms of the family, attention is not directed particularly at the formidable and complicated task of how everybody interacts with everybody else, but instead at how the family generates pressures on him or provides relief from stresses, encourages his self-confidence and autonomy or requires dependency, etc., certainly a more manageable research venture.

Some of these differences can be resolved. If the family is the focus, single individuals living alone can still be traced through the family. While a commitment exists to study the individual's mental health as a dependent variable, this does not bar the addition of other dependent variables. Shifting to the other side, if you start with the individual you can include the family constellation, perhaps by employing a shorter evaluation method for them. After all, you still want to know the characteristics of those around him, one of which is their mental health.

CRITICAL FACTORS IN FAMILY LIFE

Some of the discussion centered on the factors in family life in an urban setting that are apt to maximize the likelihood of becoming ill. Three areas of variables were identified: (1) characteristics of individuals; (2) age-sex relationships (mother-child, husband-wife, sibling-sibling, etc.); (3) extent to which the family carries out its functions. The research of Koos, who studied how families dealt with their troubles, was cited. He found that the extent to which the family was organized on certain criteria determined their success, criteria such as recognition and acceptance of each other's roles and investment in the family as an on-going institution. Caplan and Rapoport are concentrating on the standard crises in the ontogeny of the family, engagement, marriage, birth of first child, departure of last child, etc. Their attempt is to gauge the effects with a view to prior-preparation and therapeutic intervention if aid is indicated.

It was suggested that there are recurring situations in family life that lend themselves to research on the effects to individuals. One of these might be the loss of a job by the husband and when, sometimes, the wife will seek work. Another is the illness of one member, ending in death. A third could be the adjustment required upon moving into a new neighborhood. Moving further toward the standardization of stimuli, the question was raised about the fruitfulness of small group research for hypotheses on family functioning, and the possibility of employing experimental family problem-solving situations for an understanding of leadership, change in composition, communication patterns, and the location of trouble on a subsample of the family population. Another view of "standardization" was not to attempt to correlate a variety of family problems on the malfunctioning of members, but, rather, to view these more abstractly as stresses or pressures, a concept that lends itself to application across the sample.

VALUES

A study of American families regarded as successful found the basis for this judgment rested on their achievement as parents in raising children who were not delinquent and providing them with a college education. These families insulated themselves from neighbors possessing different values and made certain that those they selected as friends held similar views. The degree of congruence of values, at the community-family and the intra-family levels, has been of interest to researchers. It does present problems for people don't always do what they say they believe in, as disclosed in the work in Elmira on attitudes and performance of restaurant proprietors toward Negroes. One view taken is that the normal application of our personal value system is that we use it to assess people even if it does not reflect itself in our behavior, although in that case it may have psychic repercussions such as quiet and self-disparagement.

The divergence of expressed values and behavior also can result from a conflict of values. This is apparent currently in school integration in Berkeley, where parents with liberal civil rights views and strong feelings about the education of their children are faced with the possible deleterious effect of lowered school standards. Values imbedded in a situation involving a high degree of emotion or one encouraging socially acceptable responses may warrant projective methods. In this regard, there is a technique evolved by Ralph White who attempts to get at latent value assumptions regardless of what the person says. The rationale is that in any communication people will express their values regardless of what they say. You get at the individual's underlying value structure by the words that are used, classifying these into pre-determined categories. One participant, who has investigated this method, commented that White's categories are just a suggestion, and use would require the construction of a detailed coding manual. Instead, recourse was taken in a more judgmental way of rating fifty values comparable to a scheme devised by Sears, Maccoby, and Levin.

Several values emerged as pertinent to psychiatric disorder in the research in Stirling County. One is reported by Longaker and Cleveland in *Explorations in Social Psychiatry*. They identify it as the disparagement syndrome. "I'm no good, my family is no good, the community is no good. There's no use trying because you can't do anything about it." It amounts to a prevailing attitude that is socially self-defeating. Srole's anomie scale can be regarded as essentially consisting of disparagement items of this order. Then, there is a conflict in values, in Florence Kluckhohn's terms, between "being" and "doing." Those believing in enjoying themselves, their families, and their friends, and not earning more money than is sufficient for basic needs and reasonable security, are disparaged by others who advocate unending striving in the Calvinistic tradition. The genesis of a good deal of psychiatric disorder is lodged here. A value or sentiment that clearly distinguishes A's from D's is the quality of being able to detach oneself from stress of the environment at some point, and a concomitant ability is being able to intensely enjoy ordinary things, sunshine, even simple household tasks.

Farber's scales on parental relations with children asks in part for husbands and wives to rank from one to ten the values important to their marriage, the score being the rank order correlation. These deal with cultural values such as healthy and happy children, extent of companionship between husband and wife, the community's view of the family as stable and responsible, etc. In Aberdeen, class differences rooted in reality influenced the findings on similar measures. Asked to check from a list of 20 items the three considered most important, the lower classes stressed adequate food and clothing, while these rarely were selected in the upper brackets—where emotional factors (the child should be loved) predominated. It suggests the need for caution in recognizing bias caused by economic or ethnic divergencies in the population.

FAMILY FUNCTIONING

Basically, family functioning relates to the extent that people are effective in providing nutrients for each other, whether food or clothing or love or support. Particularly when probing emotional areas one is likely to meet with difficulty in securing reliable information. People certainly are aware of what is going on, but it is another matter to trust an interviewer not to reveal something to one's mate (who will be interviewed later), or even to "confess" face-to-face about certain unrequited needs. Feldman has developed a draw-a-family test with a number of indices that, in his opinion, are not evident to the subject. He is asked to tell stories about the drawing in relation to particular questions. Who does he put into it? Where is he? Where is the same sex person? In what order are they drawn? Another, more direct approach is to ask the respondent who the significant others in his life are (positive or negative) and probe these interactions. Also, if a person expected to be significant isn't mentioned, to find out the "why" for it. Brun sets up three problems for both parents (congruence is of interest), situations of masturbation, theft, and failure to study, and he provides six solutions for each. The parent is asked to rank order these and write down his reasons for this arrangement as well as a prognosis for each solution. Objective data is relatively easy to collect on children by means of independent school ratings in order to determine the extent to which difficulties expected do occur outside the family.

A variable of proven meaning for measurement of family functioning is its social interaction patterns, and of particular importance here for judgment of its adjustment is the extent to which it utilizes the environment. How aware is the family of the community resources, and how willing is it to use them? Does a mutually helpful neighborliness exist in the environment and is the family integrated into the system? For urban study, a more liberal evaluation of kinship ties may be indicated. The "nuclear" family in a nongeographic situation may obtain a good deal of interaction and substantial support by means of the telephone, letters, and annual events. It probably is not as "nuclear" as is supposed.

The Nova Scotia research determined certain community phenomena that were related to the prevalence of mental illness, such as lack of leadership, poor communication, etc. Are there parallels for family functioning? Koos' measures are somewhat similar—good communication between family members, complementarity of role structure, commitment of members to the family as a going concern, etc. These add up to a cohesive quality, and on this basis one might be able to spell it out in variables such as intrafamily communication patterns, participation in household tasks, degree of isolation of individual members, affection, etc. An appropriate selection, or at least to assure a sufficiently inclusive one, may be to systematically inspect the findings in other studies to determine the factors that show a strong relationship with mental illness. The heart of the matter then becomes one of determining which of these (present or absent) help the person to help himself, and the more there are the better.

Dr. Mirra Komarovsky attended the 7th meeting of the seminar and presented the findings of her recent research on blue-collar workers that had relevance to family functioning. Studies of the family have been based, for the most part, either on college-educated or middle-class segments, or on disorganized elements among the lower classes. Dr. Komarovsky's concern, in contrast, was with the stable marriage relationship in working-class families with the view toward determining the congruences and discrepancies in values and behavior among the marriage partners and the sources for the divergencies, and toward ascertaining whether generalizations made about marriage processes based on populations located at the other end of the socio-economic scale were applicable here or were class-linked.

Sixty families were studied in all. The size of the sample required certain criteria to reduce heterogeneity. Families were to be Protestant in faith, marriage partners living together, not over 40 years in age, possessing no more than a high school education, and with children. The occupation of the principal breadwinner had to qualify as "blue collar," and the preponderance of the sample were in semiskilled and skilled activities. In actuality, there were some mixed-faith marriages and a few Roman Catholic families. The respondents were obtained from a New Jersey community near Newark and were not selected on a random basis.

The marital problems of this blue-collar group, and they were considerable, do not appear to be related to the dominant theories of family disorganization, such as goal conflict or disturbances caused by ambiguities in cultural directives. Cultural consensus among husbands and wives was remarkable in terms of Farber's measure of cohesion; they knew what to expect of each other and there was little disagreement or discontent with regard to task allocation or roles in general, in contrast, for example, with the dissatisfaction expressed by college women. It appears that cultural consensus is not synonymous with social health.

The study attempted to assess psychic intimacy, disclosure and sharing, empathy, emotional support for each in the relationship, and their self-confidence outside of the marriage. Interviewing took six hours at the minimum, at least two 2-hour sessions with the wife and one 2-hour session with the husband: It was guided, with a few scales, many test stories, and open questions. A characteristic finding was a certain absence of institutional conflict, for the mother usually was the guide for the young couple in the early years of the marriage, the same agency that fashioned their expectations in adolescence. The main difficulty, according to Dr. Komarovsky, is that the norms of marriage are dysfunctional for marriage adjustment, the fault lying in the structural conditions of life, and aggravated by a discrepancy between the couple's aspirations and the opportunity for actual attainment.

Despite the attempt at homogeneity, the data disclosed two subgroups based on the extent of education, workers who had not completed high school (40 families), and those that had completed it. While the latter had similar occupations, they did earn a little more money and were closer to middle class in their ideals, etc.

Among the less educated (not high school graduates), the feeling was strong that marriage meant mutual devotion, cooperation in family tasks, and sexual rapport. But they found friendship difficult to achieve with the opposite sex. Women were more apt to discuss intimate things with other women, while men felt their wives were not interested in what interested them; as a consequence they had little to say to each other. Besides this gap in interests, among men there existed a strong feeling that the expressing of emotions was unmanly. They were likely to withdraw in times of tension and find solace in physical activity rather than social interaction, although this reaction could be interspersed by violent outbreaks.

The more educated blue-collar worker (high school graduate) shares more of his experiences with his wife and knows more about what is going on in her world. The less educated one in the interview had much less to say about himself. It was not only a matter of articulateness, it also was a selective reserve. He admitted feelings of anger easily, but not hurt, his model of masculinity being that one doesn't talk about such things, and it results in a sharp break with the feminine world.

There are some satisfactory marriages that work out this way under certain conditions. The requirement is the presence of others to supply each function that is not provided in the marriage, such as the extended family, friends, a male clique, and it will work. The difficulty is great when the family is isolated from a network of relatives and friends. This is increasingly true these days with the rise in geographic mobility as people go where the work is available. It is a different mobility than one generated by social or career aspirations. Participation in groups is minimal and the result is an immense amount of physical togetherness in the marriage in the absence of other affiliations. The wife sits alone, and she is lonely if he's out, or if he's in and bored.

The circumstances of lower socio-economic class marriages in Aberdeen was related for comparison. Courtship is brief, wedlock and conception comes early: the period of leaving school and being an independent adult being a short one, two or three years on the average. With the housing shortage, 60 to 70 percent of newlyweds begin married life in the parent's home (usually the girl's), and it continues until after the birth of the first and sometimes the second child. The child is as much a child of the grandparents as of the parents, especially if the wife continues to work. When the family is rehoused, and if it is in another part of the city, at the most it cannot be more than half an hour away. A check made five years after the birth of the first child showed that the wife in a third of the families saw her mother or another family member five times a week. The husband only participates in this activity on weekends when he and his family visit his parents. Families do exist that have moved and are divorced from their extended kin because of tragedy or conflict, but not as a result of upward mobility. Like the population of the research under discussion, they are thrown very much on their own resources.

One view expressed was that what appeared to be happening here was that a relationship designed for one set of circumstances did not work out well when these were changed. For long periods of time, marriages with this expectation of intimacy, or lack of it, were arranged by parents and defined and approved by society as the appropriate behavior, and they resulted in stable relationships.

In Czechoslovskia, as an example, prior to the war, when the young farmer married, he and his wife decided that the yard and poultry were her domain, the field and stock his. She had charge of the children, except for the boys when they were old enough to work in the fields. This kept the couple from having to share in decisions, and except for bed and meals, when the family was together, they had no contact. After the evening meal the farmer retreated to the pub and his cronies, while his wife sat around with other women, embroidering, pulling feathers, gossiping and telling stories, while the children clustered around and listened. This situation was institutionalized. It appears to have been a defense against being thrown together too much while having to live closely the rest of their lives; as if to do away with individuality so that idiosyncrasies of personality would have as little influence as possible in the relationship. This arrangement, it was pointed out, is found in widely dispersed areas such as Japan, in the Arctic among Eskimos, in Scotland in remote places, and in Ireland among the country people.

It would seem that a familiar style of marriage among the population under scrutiny is in process of change. New expectations do emerge but there are no facilities for their realization. Joint decision-making is accepted, the authority of the women is considerable, yet the achievement of a companionate style of marriage is remote for them. It is not only the women who are lonely; a growing isolation goes on among the men as their relations with other men tend to weaken between the ages of 30 and 40. In fact, the women maintain their early contacts more. Among the group, very little social life in couples occurs.

These blue-collar marriages appear to be located somewhere between the formalization of the relationship illustrated by the Czech farm family and an informal kind which stresses closeness, support, and participation. In contrast to the minimal demands on each other made in the cultures of arranged marriages, the stress here, aided by movies and television, is toward maximal interrelatedness. The marriages in question probably are acutely impoverished without the supports that make the formal type tenable or the emotional maturity required by the greater intimacy.

An investigation of the role of women in Nigeria, where polygamy is practiced, found that rural women coped with their condition by stressing the importance of rearing young children during most of the life cycle. Urban women, educated in Christian schools, with an expectation of monogamous companionate marriage were more dissatisfied with their lot.

The question was raised as to whether there are pathological consequences. Does it make a difference for the mental health of those individuals who are involved? The research was not aimed at determining this, but it did record that among the men the atmosphere is one of anti-intraperception, an unwillingness to look inside; a view that this is a feminine thing and part of the complex of emotions that they attempt to deny. One investigator has suggested that it may be a strong feminine identification, perhaps caused by role segregation in the raising of children, that the male child later grapples with by overemphasizing his masculinity. The women were more dissatisfied than the men, but neither one thought in mental health terms. Almost no probing of motives takes place, not because of the lack of curiosity, but rather that they had no concepts to meet it. Yet the psychiatrist was a known figure and disturbed people were located in the sample. The greater discontent evidenced by women might be explained by the fact that women usually have more investment in the marriage, but here it proved to be the sole emotional relationship for the men, too. Involvement in the job was minimal and fewer of them had close relationships in comparison with women.

These marriages can be viewed as dysfunctional insofar as they do not provide for certain affiliative needs in an environment where substitutes are not available. The effect of this on the individual would depend, of course, on the strength of his need for affiliation. The overt evidence of greater dissatisfaction among women could be that the men have been conditioned for less companionship, but it is difficult to determine whether it is this or that the men are incapable of admitting the need. Men drink more, and are under other strains. For instance, they are ambivalent about their women going to work to supplement the family income, because they are jealous of their wives' association with other men and are challenged about their abilities as an economic provider. It caused them anxiety because their position is difficult to justify with bills to be paid and other advantages, and because of the selfishness patent in his attitude, since the man would be saddled with some of his wife's responsibilities when their working hours dovetailed.

Earlier the claim was made that there was a consensus among husbands and wives concerning the marriage norms. The fault lay in the absence of the supports requisite for this type of marriage to adequately function. An alternative hypothesis is that it could be a conflict of norms and not a consensus, with the women having an expectation radically different than the one held by the men. This appeared to be so in some cases, but by and large although loneliness was expressed by the women, indignation was not. The husband was not viewed as in the wrong; the less educated were likely to say, "What's more natural than a man like this."

Another alternative explanation could be along an isolation-nonisolation dimension. The woman by virtue of her role as housekeeper and mother is alone at home a good deal of the day, while the man has a certain amount of social interaction with other adults at his place of work. The loneliness expressed by the wife might be the result of this inevitable isolation. But the women were not completely alone, they had other women as confidantes. Besides, a clue appears in answer to a question posed in the interview. Men, when asked about their preference as favorite associate on a list of activities of interest to them, specified their wives more frequently in activities of secondary interest compared to what they were most interested in doing. The wives, for their part, desired their husbands most as partners for their prime activities.

A question was raised that deals with the identification of loneliness as the crucial aspect in the marital relationship. When answering what is felt to be lacking, the woman may be stating the aspect she is least satisfied with, but this is not necessarily the most important thing in the absolute hierarchy of the person. In rebuttal, it is claimed that the loneliness interpretation has support in a comparison of findings for the more and the less educated groups. Those who have finished high school are experiencing more sharing and the use of each other for emotional support, and express less dissatisfaction with their marriages than those who did not complete their high school education.

A possible bias here between what is, in effect, a class comparison, is that the less educated simply may have less to talk about, that they suffer from an impoverishment in their environment. It may well be that the higher the education level the more likely it is that people will have stimulating contact with others and more to discuss. The measure employed for determining the extent of sharing was a compilation of an inventory of experiences over the past two weeks and determining whether it had been discussed with the marriage partner. Impoverishment undoubtedly existed; in the interview the less educated displayed less ability to take the role of the interviewee: They reported in a flat manner with little emotion or sophistication.

Impoverishment in disclosure can be a reaction to the interviewer's own background. It does appear that these two groups differ in their cultural distance from the observer. The statement was offered that some reservation did exist about the interview situation with men, but this was because the interviewers were women and not because of their class. One of the interviewers was extremely at ease with the women and her protocols were richer in content than the other two. The type of intimate information that was revealed about sexual life, resentments toward the husband, etc., does seem to indicate an absence of reserve. In research in Nova Scotia, concern was felt on a parallel problem, but information from other sources, such as key informants well-acquainted with the respondents and participant observers, led to the conclusion that if the individuals in question had a richer inner life than they revealed, they were masters at concealing it.

The findings in this research emphasize the sensitivity of communication patterns as a measurement of family relationships. The type of communication investigated was concerned with companionship. Is there a difference between it and the kind that is related to family functioning? Separation or distinction between instrumental and emotional content in communication would seem to present difficulty since they can be indistinguishable. Talking about the children or grocery bills is a way, too, of expressing one's feelings toward another. It must be kept in mind that communication is essential where roles are shared, but not nearly so where they are highly segregated. Another qualification is not to ignore other methods than verbal response. Class and cultural differences may be reflected in the extent of recourse to, for instance, physical gestures.

Note: Dr Chein extracted a number of dimensions of family cohesiveness that were implied or explicitly stated during the discussion. These are listed below:

Some Dimensions of Family Cohesiveness
by ISIDOR CHEIN, Ph.D.

1. Preference for one another's company over company of others.

2. Frequency of occasions for togetherness.

3. Absence of sense of constraint to togetherness (e.g., absence of dispersal as soon as formalities are over).

4. Absence of interpersonal rivalry, hostility, contrient interdependence. (Note: A and B are contriently interdependent if A's achievement of his goals interferes with B's achievement of his goals, and vice versa).

5. Absence of shifting intrafamilial coalitions and/or permanent factions.

6. Presence of promotive interdependence.

7. (Note: A and B are promotively interdependent if A's achievement of his goals facilitates B's achievement of his goals and vice versa.)

7. Voluntary extension of personal life space into family arena (e.g., vicarious sharing of personal experiences; mutuality of consultation and advice-seeking on personal problems; invitation of others to extrafamilial recreational activities).

8. Acceptance of restrictions for sake of others (e.g., in determination of TV programs when a particular member has a strong desire for a particular program; taking on of anothers' chores when they are tired, overworked, pressed for time; quietness and considerateness when others are ill, sleeping, studying, in need of solitude; tolerance of others when they are out-of-sorts; etc.).

9. Mobilization in face of threat to members.

10. Deviancy of cohesiveness pattern from modal patterns of social stratum and community.

8

The Family Setting

HAROLD FELDMAN, Ph.D. AND LLOYD A. BRIGHTMAN, Ph.D.

INTRODUCTION

The family as a setting for the shaping of social behavior is of obvious importance. Very few members of society escape its influence, and for each one it is the first, if not the most powerful, social force encountered, preparing the stage for all future development. Because of its priority and intensity, the socialization experienced within the family interacts with all later experience.

Despite its central position, the importance of the family sometimes fails to be reflected in the literature. One reason for this is the diverse nature of family research. A review of family literature reveals a variety of approaches employed in an attempt to delineate its nature and function. Family theory has been characterized by Nye and Berardo [1] as "an intellectual enterprise (which does not define) what is being attempted . . . with a number of scholars commencing from different points, with different intellectual tools and somewhat different objectives."

In a very real sense there is no family theory as such. As

[1] Nye, F., & Berardo, F. *Emerging conceptual frameworks in family analysis.* New York: The McMillan Co., 1966.

Christensen [2] has pointed out, many researchers seem to stop short at the point of developing propositions, without integrating them into the over-all principles demanded by a theory. He assigns this as a major cause for "the unfortunate eclecticism that has characterized the family field of study."

FAMILY CONCEPTUAL FRAMEWORKS

While there may be no theory, implications for theory or theories exist in a number of different conceptual frameworks, as that term is used by Hill and Hansen [3], Zetterberg [4], and Nye and Berardo [1] to indicate clusters of essential concepts and the assumptions upon which they rest. Lacking the precision of a theory, a conceptual framework is, nevertheless, a necessary condition for theory building.

The conceptual frameworks dealing with the family divide themselves into four broad groups: those derived from sociology; those having their roots in idiosyncratic psychology; those with a social-psychological focus; and those influenced by the developmental approach. Each of these differs in the perspective from which the family is viewed and, as a result, the kinds of variables considered. A close look at these four broad areas, and typical research studies that each has produced, may serve to throw into relief some of the difficulties facing this field of study and to highlight some of the promise each holds, not only for researchers in family, but for social scientists dealing with other problem areas.

A major goal of social science is to interrelate information gained

[2] Christensen, H. *Normative theory derived from cross-cultural research.* Working Paper Number 17, Institute for the Study of Social Change, Department of Sociology, Purdue University, 1968 (mimeograph).
[3] Hill, R., & Hansen, D. The identification of conceptual frameworks utilized in family study. *Marriage and Family Living*, 1960, 22, 299-311.
[4] Zetterberg, H. *On theory and verification.* Totowa, N.J.: The Bedminister Press., Inc., 1965.

through research. An example of this may be found in Leighton's hypothesis relating community disintegration to the prevalence of psychiatric disorder (developed elsewhere in this volume). The present paper attempts this function by discussing each of the conceptual frameworks in terms of concepts important for the family, and by developing the implications of these for Leighton's hypothesis.

Sociological Frameworks

The sociological approaches to family studies divide into two major groups: those viewing the family as an institution, and those stressing the structural-functional aspects of the family and the implications of these for society. While some overlap between these two focuses exists, there are enough differences in emphasis to consider them separate research areas [1, 5].

In the first group, the relationship of the family to other social institutions is of central concern. A social institution consists in the routinizing of rules and roles without which society cannot sustain itself. Thus, the common defense is assured by the institution of government; the problem of the distribution of goods necessary for existence is solved by that of the economy; relatively consistent behavior is partly achieved by the institution of religion.

The family, when viewed as an institution, becomes with these an instrument of social control, being responsible for the replacing of lost members and, along with the educational institution, for the socialization of new members. However, other institutions influence the family and are influenced by it, giving rise to the dynamic quality of society.

[5] Christensen, H. Development of the family field of study. In Harold T. Christensen (Ed.) *Handbook of marriage and the family*. Chicago: Rand McNally & Co., 1964, Pp. 3-32.

As may be imagined, where the unit of interest is the institution, rather than some more narrowly defined entity, research studies employing the institutional approach have tended to be more descriptive than analytical, and as Kenkel [6] points out, focuses on "the idea of the family rather than on the internal workings of particular family groups." Several analyses have attempted to show that family structure is culturally determined [7, 8]. Others have recognized the effect of the family upon society [9, 10]. Certain particular variables of interest do emerge, however. Among them are the stability of the family and effects of social milieu upon the marital dyad and upon child-rearing.

Research done by Miller and Swanson [11] and Edwards [12] illustrate the institutional approach focused upon particular family variables. In the first, families were classified according to two ideal types, entrepreneurial and bureaucratic. Tracing the changes that occurred as a result of the shift from small business (entrepreneurial) to big corporations (bureaucratic) and concomitant changes in role needs, they then compared child-rearing practices of the two groups. They found that entrepreneurial parents tended to be more strict and achievement oriented, while bureaucratic parents were more other-directed and permissive, tending more to adjustment in their child-rearing.

[6] Kenkel, W. *The family in perspective*. New York: Appleton, Century, Crofts, Inc., 1960.
[7] Queen, S. & Adams, J. *The family in various culture*. Philadelphia: Lippincott, 1952.
[8] Sirjamaki, J. Cultural configurations in the American family. *American Journal of Sociology*, 1948, 53, 467-470.
[9] Zimmerman, C. *Family and civilization*. New York: Harper & Row, Publishers, 1947.
[10] Mimkoff, M. (Ed.) *Comparative family systems*. Boston: Houghton Mifflin Co., 1965.
[11] Miller, D., & Swanson, G. *The changing American parent*. New York: John Wiley, 1958.
[12] Edwards, H. Black Muslim and Negro Christian family relationships. *Journal of Marriage and the Family*, 1968, 30, 604-610.

Edwards, in a comparison of fourteen matched pairs of families, examined differences between those affiliated with the Nation of Islam (Muslim) and those who held membership in Negro Christian churches, in the specific areas of husband-wife relationships, extended-family relationships, and parent-child relationships. The results indicate that Muslim families, in comparison to Christian families, tend to typify middle-class ideals with respect to sex practices, value placed on education, industriousness, and interest in developing mental and physical alertness. Not only were Muslims more conforming, but "there exists a narrower gap between . . . ideational values and their normative behavior."

In the second major group of studies employing the sociological approach, we find those that represent earlier efforts in the family field, making use of historical and/or cross-cultural methods to analyze family organization, often in its connection with broader kinship groups. Studies of this sort tend to be comparative, focusing upon such areas of interest as marriage types, family formation, rules of residence, descent, and family authority. (For numerous examples, see Refs. [13] and [14].)

This group is dominated, however, by studies under the rubric of structural-functional analysis. Here attempts are made to outline the range and importance of the various functions fulfilled by the family for the individual and for society. Examples of research areas here include effects of technology upon family structure, social class differences, and the relationship between the family and the educational system. This approach assumes that certain functional requirements must be met in order for a social group to survive at a given level. These requirements are met by subsystems, of which the

[13] Linton, R. *The study of man*. New York: Appleton-Century-Crofts, Inc., 1936.
[14] Murdock, G. *Social structure*. New York: The Free Press, 1949.

family is one. In turn, the family has its own functional requirements comparable to those of larger groups. It further assumes that social systems perform individual-serving functions as well as society-serving functions.

Three important relationships stand out from these assumptions. The first focuses upon the functions that the family performs for the larger social group, e.g., replacement of members of society lost through death, and the socialization of these new members. Research regarding this relationship is interesting for its failure to agree upon the universality of any one family function. Spiro [15], for example, points out that in the kibbutz the family has lost both its socialization function and its economic function. (See also Refs. [16] and [17].)

The second relationship to emerge from the assumptions of structural-functional analysis deals with the functions of the subsystems within the family, for the family and each other. Here attention is focused on the interrelatedness of the various dyads—husband-wife, parent-child, sibling-sibling. Many studies concerned with the functionality of one subsystem for another have investigated the effects of the division of labor within the family group upon family structure. Many of them have built upon the thinking of Parsons and Bales [18], who emphasize the importance of instrumental-expressive role differentiation. (See also Refs. [19] and [20].) Zelditch [21], for example,

[15] Spiro, M. Is the family universal? The Israeli case. In N. W. Bell and E. F. Vogel (Eds.) *A Modern Introduction to the Family*. New York: Free Press of Glencoe, Inc., 1960.

[16] Gough, E. The Nayars and the definition of marriage. *Journal of Royal; Anthropological Institute*, 1959, 89, 23-34.

[17] Levy, M., & Fallers, L. The family: Some comparative considerations. *American Anthropologist*. 1959, 61, 647-651.

[18] Parsons, T., & Bales, R. *Family, socialization and interaction process.* Glencoe, Ill.: The Free Press, 1955.

[19] Slater, P. Parental role differentiation. *American Journal of Sociology*, 1961, 67, 296-308.

[20] Blake, J. *Family structure in Jamaica: the social context of reproduction.* New York: Free Press of Glencoe, Inc., 1961.

[21] Zelditch, M., Jr. Role differentiation in the nuclear family: a comparative

sampled fifty-six societies for which data was available and found that forty-six of them displayed the Parsons-Bales role structure, with the husband-father occupying the instrumental role and the wife-mother the expressive.

The third relationship concerns the consequences of family functions for the personality development of the individual. Typical of studies focusing on this aspect is an investigation by Strodtbeck [22] of achievement motivation in Jewish and Italian youths. Here, what appeared at first to be marked differences in the achievement motive due to ethnic group membership disappeared when socio-economic status was controlled for.

Certain important hypotheses emerge from this over-view of sociological frameworks as they relate to the field of family study. These may be summarized as follows: (1) societies are made up of institutions that are functionally interrelated; (2) institutions are themselves made up of subsystems that are functionally interrelated; (3) the family is an institution that is functionally interrelated subsystems. Implicit in these hypotheses is the notion that society determines in broad terms what shall constitute an effective family. It may vary in structural detail from culture to culture, but always, in order for society to maintain itself at a given level, it must conform to certain cultural imperatives.

Buckley [23] has characterized society as "a complex adaptive system ... open 'internally' as well as externally in that the interchanges among (its) components may result in significant changes in the nature of the components themselves." It is in this characteristic of

study. In T. Parsons and R. Bales (Eds.) *Family, socialization and interaction process*. New York: Free Press of Glencoe, Inc., 1955.
[22] Strodbeck, F. Family interaction, values, and achievement. In David C. McClelland et al. (Eds.) *Talent and society*. Princeton, N.J.: Van Nostrand Co., Inc., 1958.
[23] Buckley, W. Society as a complex adaptive system. In Walter Buckley (Ed.) *Modern systems research for the social scientist*. Chicago: Aldine Publishing Co., 1968, Pp. 490-513.

adaptive (as opposed to equilibrial) systems that we find an important implication for Leighton's hypothesis, using the perspective employed by the sociological framework of the family.

(1) Social institutions are interrelated so that modification of one results in modification of others.

(2) On the broad interinstitutional level, the tensions resulting under the impact of wide-spread poverty, cultural confusion, and excessive secularization (indices used by Leighton to measure degree of community disintegration), would interfere with the family's capacity to fulfill its functions.

(3) There is a reciprocal effect so that when family functions are not performed for the larger society, a more disintegrated community results.

Examples that come immediately to mind spring from important issues that are currently plaguing society. Prominent among these is the American Negro family, with its significant shift from male to female as occupier of the instrumental role, and the comparatively recent dramatic changes in *normative* sexual behavior among young adults.

Frameworks Based on Idiosyncratic Psychology

Where the sociological frameworks orient themselves toward society, regarding the individual as a product of an impersonal culture that exists before his birth, molds his development through various social devices, and continues after his death, idiosyncratic psychology focuses directly upon the individual, specifically upon his intrapsychic nature and the modifications it undergoes under the impact of personal experience.

Students of idiosyncratic psychology owe most of their heritage to Freud, who postulated three basic components whose interaction made up human personality: the id—the unconscious, primitive aspects of human personality that serve as the source for all psychic energy; the ego—that component of the personality that represents reality as the actor perceives it; and the super-ego—made up of conscience, derived from parental prohibitions, and ego ideal, based on parental approval and representing the self as he would like to be.

From this it is apparent that a basic assumption of idiosyncratic psychology is the belief that personality is not inborn, but rather the product of one's earliest experiences within the family. In general, this point of view argues that the development of values and socialization are parallel and interdependent processes, beginning in infancy when the child lives within the mother's sphere of values. The child's eventual progress away from an exclusive relationship with the mother to relationships with other family members is a critical step deeply influenced by the quality of the earlier relationship and by the conditions under which the break in that exclusive union is made. A traumatic rupture, it is theorized, sets the stage for identity crises; a gradual growing away from the mother that is free from stress permits the ever-broadening relationships required of the adult.

Along with an identity established for oneself within the family environment, there develops a value orientation. As one writer puts it [24], "the psychic center of gravity for the individual is this identity and a corresponding set of standards, strivings, and values." As the individual moves out into new groups beyond the family, these values undergo changes in response to changes in social needs. The successful resolution of the conflict inevitably accompanying the necessity to modify one's values can contribute to growth and mental health. If the struggle with conflict fails, however, the result is adaptive breakdown.

With the successful resolution of value conflicts, the individual achieves a stage of maturity that permits him to form meaningful relationships with others in his social group. Referred to variously as

[24] Ackerman, N. *The psychodynamics of family life*. New York: Basic Books, 1958.

"ego integration" [25], "self-actualization" [26], "productive" [27], or "fully functioning" [28], this stage represents the acme of individual development and, as the terms implies, permits the individual to contribute to his social group in the most efficient way, unhampered by unresolved internal conflict.

Given this configuration of concepts with which to view the individual, studies employing this framework have dealt with a number of different variables—the Oedipus complex, needs, personality types, unconscious motivation, libido, and cathexis. These concepts, and others, have been applied to a wide range of family problems, including mate selection, distribution of authority, marital conflict and marital disintegration, interspousal communication, deviant sexual practices, and personality fulfillment within marriage.

Because of difficulties in operationalizing many of the variables pertinent to the framework of idiosyncratic psychology, research findings in this area tend to be less than definitive and are often open to alternative interpretations. Christensen [5] dismisses it as a framework for family study since it "focuses upon the individual rather than upon the family per se." Komarovsky and Waller [29], however, maintain that it "tends always to explain the behavior of the adult in terms of his previous experience in the parental family . . . ."

Sears [30] has reviewed over 150 reports of various investigations employing concepts deriving from idiosyncratic psychology. Orlan-

[25] Erikson, E. *Childhood and society*. New York: W.W. Norton & Co., Inc., 1950.
[26] Maslow, A. *Motivation and personality*. New York: Harper & Brothers, Publishers, 1954.
[27] Fromm, E. *Man for himself*. New York: Holt, Rinehart & Winston, 1947.
[28] Rodgers, C. *Client-centered therapy*. New York: Houghton Mifflin Co., 1951.
[29] Komarovsky, M., & Waller, W. Studies of the family. *American Journal of Sociology*, 1945, 50, 443-451.
[30] Sears, R. Survey of objective studies of psychoanalytic concepts. *Social Science Research Bulletin*, 1943, 51.

sky [31] has also reviewed an equal number of studies concerning the relationship between child care and subsequent personality development. Sewell [32] studied 162 farm children in an attempt to establish a relationship between child-rearing practices and subsequent personality development. He was unable to do so.

Although not supported by research, Kenkel [6] has employed the concept of Oedipal attachment to explain mate selection: "Some individuals carry their Oedipal attachment to adulthood and seem compelled to fall in love with and marry someone who resembles their parent. It is as if the only person psychologically suited as a mate is the parent of the opposite sex" (p. 443).

Winch (1952), drawing heavily upon ideas of both Freudian and non-Freudian writers, has developed a theory of love based on needs. He proposed two kinds of "complementariness" that would attract marriage partners to each other: where one is high and the other low with respect to the same need; and where the partners exhibit different, but complementary, needs. Given appropriate socio-cultural conditions, e.g., marriage culturally defined as gratifying, based on free choice of partners, and sufficient opportunity for premarital interaction, an individual would select his marital partner, through unconscious motivation, upon the basis of unsatisfied needs within his own personality.

In order to validate his theory, Winch interviewed, simultaneously and separately, twenty-five young couples who had been married less than two years. A Thematic Apperception Test was administered to each one in the sample, in addition to the questionnaires that served as the basis for the interview. A correlational analysis of the data supported the complementarity of needs notion. Sixty-six percent of

[31] Orlansky, H. Infant care and personality. *Psychological Bulletin,* 1949, **46,** 1-48.
[32] Sewell, W. Infant training and the personality of the child. *American Journal of Sociology,* 1952, 58, 150-159.

the predicted correlations showed the hypothesized sign. In a more recent paper [33], Winch has answered criticism of his work with a re-analysis of the same data, offering the same degree of support.

Several relationships of importance between the family and Leighton's hypothesis emerge from a consideration of the frameworks based on idiosyncratic psychology:

(1) The fulfillment of self, especially the capacity for forming meaningful relationships with others, is a function of one's earliest intrafamilial experiences.

(2) Effective family functioning is indexed by the extent to which it provides a milieu permitting the development of this capacity.

(3) Failure to develop the self results in less effective functioning beyond the boundaries of the family.

(4) An integrated society provides channels through which family members can move toward self-fulfillment.

Where the sociological approach views the family as a subsystem of society in a functional relationship with other subsystems, the approach of idiosyncratic psychology would evaluate a society according to the ability of its members to relate to each other.

There is much in idiosyncratic psychology that speaks directly to Leighton's hypothesis concerning community disintegration and the prevalence of psychiatric disorder, since intrapsychic factors are the central concern of this approach. Just as a child identifies with his parents, members of a social group must identify with it by incorporating the dominant ethics of the group into their own self-structures. If a parent fails to offer security to a child, the child neither identifies with, nor conforms to, the ethics of the parent.

On a societal level, a disintegrated community, where norms are shifting and not clearly set, would offer little security to its members, and it would therefore be hazardous for members to accept its ethical

[33] Winch, R. Another look at the theory of complementary needs in mate-selection. *Journal of Marriage and the Family*, 1967, 29, 756-762.

standards and unprofitable to conform. Further, it would work against
the family's ability to achieve self-fulfillment for its members.
Self-fulfillment is predicated upon the satisfaction of more basic needs.
The effects of an environment that failed to do this would be as
deleterious for family development as a family environment of this sort
would be for the development of the individual.

Conversely, an individual who has been unable to develop the
capacity to relate to others within the family will be unable to relate to
others within the broader social group. This leads us once again to the
idea of interaction between the family and society.

Social-Psychological Frameworks

The social-psychological view of the family represents approaches
intermediate to the sociological and the idiosyncratic psychological, by
looking on the family as a "unity of interacting personalities [34].
Included in this general area are the interactionist approach, the
situational approach, and exchange theory. It is probably true that
these social-psychological frameworks have been most important for
shifting the emphasis in family study from a broad institutional
orientation to a direct focus upon the internal workings of the family as
individual family members interact.

Prominent among the social-psychological approaches is the interactionist framework. It differs from those previously considered in
several important ways: unlike idiosyncratic psychology, it gives little
thought to unconscious processes; unlike the structural-functional
approach, it considers family relationships to be in a constant state of
flux rather than in equilibrium. Moreover, it holds that behavior is
largely derived from communication processes and that social objects

[34] Burgess, E. The family as a unity of interacting personalities. *The Family*,
1926, 7, 3-9.

are interpreted by individual family members and have a special meaning for each. Social objects, then, are not physical stimuli in the ordinary sense, but symbolic definitions of situations that assist in the process of role-taking, a concept central to this approach.

A role may be defined as a pattern of consistent behavior regulated by the norms associated with a given social position. Roles also involve clusters of values and interpretations that nelp to guide an individual's behavior in specific situations. Role-taking is the anticipation of another's response in a specific situation and modification of behavior as a result of this anticipation. (Thus, one explains tardiness to one's employer in a different manner than onc does to one's wife!) Through repetition of this process, the individual is able to organize his own behavior into a consistent pattern and to assume a position within a group.

Any position usually carries with it a number of roles that can be dominant or recessive, but always related to other reciprocal roles. A man, for example, can carry out the role of father in a father-son relationship and the role of employee in an employer-employee relationship.

Stryker [35] sums up the interactionist view of behavior by pointing out that it is premised on a classified world. One learns, through interaction, how to classify objects—including other individuals—and how to behave toward them. The meaning of the classifications one constructs resides in the shared expectations for behavior that the classifications invoke. Further, individual group members classify each other according to positions in the group structure, these classifications once again carrying with them shared expectations. This process also applies to one's identification of oneself [36], creating internalized

[35] Stryker, S. Identity salience and role performance: The relevance of symbolic interaction theory for family research. *Journal of Marriage and Family*, 1968, 30, 558-564.
[36] Mead, G. *Mind, self, and society*. Chicago: The University of Chicago Press, 1934.

expectation of one's own behavior. By constant communication, through interaction, behavior is produced and modified.

The interactionist orientation has had an important impact on family study, dating back to Burgess [34], and it has been used to investigate such topics as dating, mate selection, parent-child relationships, marital adjustment, and personality development. Its versatility has led to a preponderance of interactional studies in the total body of family research. Several studies have focused upon the family in crisis, using the interactional approach [37-39]. Employing various techniques, attempts were made to assess family stability under adverse conditions. Dyer [40] investigated the relationship of interacting units in the family and adjustment to death and birth. Using employment of the mother as an independent variable, Nye investigated the adjustment of adolescent children in the family.

A second conceptual framework involves the study of the situations to which behavior is a response. Summarized by Carr [41], the purposes of the situational approach are to break down any situation into its component elements and processes; to determine and measure the relationships among the problem phenomena, the situation, and its conditioning variables; and to discover "invariant" uniformities in co-existing relationships and in phases and trends. Some basic assumptions, as outlined by Bossard and Boll [42], indicate differences distinguishing this approach from that of the interactionist: a social situation exists as an objective, separate reality and may be studied as

[37] Angell, R. *The family encounters the depression.* New York: Charles Scribner's Sons, 1936.
[38] Koos, E. *Families in trouble.* New York: Columbia University Press, 1946.
[39] Hill, R. *Families under stress.* New York: Harper & Row, Publishers, 1949.
[40] Dyer, E. Parenthood as crises. A re-study. *Marriage and Family Living,* 1963, 25, 196-201.
[41] Carr, L. *Situational analysis: An observational approach to introductory sociology.* New York: Harper & Row, Publishers, 1948.
[42] Bossard, J., & Boll, E. *Family situations.* Philadelphia: University of Pennsylvania Press, 1943.

such; the unit of focus in a social situation is a specific human organism; a change in the basic unit of focus changes the entire situation; and each social situation is the result of the interaction of social, physical, and cultural elements.

Research studies that have employed the situational approach include Bossard and Boll [43], Blood [44], Bonilla [45], and Queen [46].

A third social-psychological framework is represented by Homans' exchange theory [47]. This attempts to describe social interaction in terms of the exchange of valued activities. He offers a set of explanatory propositions that owe much to behavioral psychology and elementary economics. Like other approaches discussed so far, it has had frequent applications to social levels beyond the family, but it is particularly applicable to that system.

Exchange theory envisages social behavior as a function of its "pay-off," varying in amount and kind depending upon the amount and kind of reward it receives. Homans' propositions are reminiscent of hypotheses dealing with reinforcement: the more often within a period of time one rewards the activity of another, the more likely he is to emit that activity; the more valuable to a man the unit of activity another gives him, the more often he will emit activity rewarded by the activity of the other; or a man in an exchange relationship with another will expect the rewards of each to be proportionate to his costs.

Several studies have made use of these principles in examining various

[43] *Ibid.* P. 47.
[44] Blood, R. A situational approach to the study of permissiveness in childrearing. *American Sociological Review*, 1953, 18, 84-87.
[45] Bonilla, E. The normative patterns of the Peurto Rican family in various situational contexts. *Dissertation Abstracts*, 1958, 18, 18-86.
[46] Queen, S. *A study of conflict situations*. Publication of the American Society, 1930, 24, 57-64.
[47] Homans, G. *Social behavior: Its elementary forms*. New York: Harcourt, Brace and World, 1961.

aspects of family life. Cancian [48], for example, has employed them to analyze the position of the mother-in-law in Mexican peasant families, showing that her power varied as a result of several factors which, in effect, governed the amount of rewards she could distribute. Bernard [49] has applied exchange principles to the development of marital adjustment patterns, generating models for interpreting and understanding this relationship.

In an investigation of the development of the husband and wife relationship, Feldman [50] found an effect which invites interpretation by exchange theory. In families where the wife had significantly more education than her husband, the husband had more decision-making power with respect to the frequency of sexual intercourse than the wife. The opposite was true in marriages where the husband's education was equal to or greater than his wife's.

Important relationships between the family and Leighton's hypothesis, inherent in the social-psychological frameworks, revolve around the ideas that:

(1) Man lives in a symbolic as well as physical environment.

(2) One learns the symbols of his environment through interaction with others, specifically, members of his family.

(3) Clusters of symbols have the effect of defining social roles.

(4) Effective fulfillment of family roles depends in large measure upon the quality of the social context and the opportunities it provides for equitable exchange relationships.

Viewed from this perspective, the family's effectiveness is judged by the competence with which the various familial positions are filled.

[48] Cancian, F. The effect of patrilocal households on nuclear family interaction in Zinacantan. *E studio de Cultura Maya*, 1965, 5, 299-315.
[49] Bernard, J. The adjustment of married mates. In H. T. Christensen (Ed.) *Handbook of marriage and the family*. Chicago: Rand McNally & Co., 1964, Pp. 675-739.
[50] Feldman, H. The development of the husband-wife relationships. Ithaca, N.Y.: Cornell University, 1961 (mimeograph).

Upon this depends the level of communication essential for teaching new members symbolic meanings of the social objects with which they come in contact. Upon this also depends the degree of integration of the family, and ultimately the integration of society.

Application of social-psychological approaches to Leighton's hypothesis demonstrates again the variety of vantage points from which one can view a given social problem. In terms of the interactional framework, a key element in disintegration would consist in the number of shared expectations available in the environment. A reduction in shared expectations would be directly related to a decrease in normative behavior. The situational approach would emphasize that social situations have an emergent quality, that is, a "reality beyond that of its component parts" [3]. Thus, the focus would shift to disintegration as a social situation capable of shaping behavior, leading to a higher degree of disintegration.

Exchange theorists would predict that the inconsistent reinforcement, or high negative reinforcement, offered by a disintegrated environment would inhibit adaptive behavior. Profits, as it were, would be reduced, influencing individual actors to drop out of exchange relationships (i.e., social interaction). This would further exacerbate the disintegrative qualities of the environment.

The Developmental Framework

Up to this point we have considered three broad approaches to family study representing a continuum leading from a focus upon society and the effects of social structure upon the structure and processes of the family (sociological), through a focus upon the interaction between social situations and the development of the family as a group of interacting personalities (social-psychological), to a focus upon the development of the individual and the implications of this for the family and society (idiosyncratic psychological).

We come now to an approach that is unique in family studies, in that it has been "consciously formulated in advance of the research it seeks to do" [5]. It is the youngest, and in many ways, the most fruitful conceptual framework to be applied to the family. As outlined by Hill and Hansen [3], it is not a unique approach, but rather a joining together of various theoretical aspects of sociology, psychology, and other family analytical approaches. In essence, this approach views the family as a semiclosed system (in that it is neither wholly dependent upon society nor wholly independent from it) of interacting personalities.

Its primary focus is upon the longitudinal career of the family system rather than the static analysis of the family at one point in time. In this way, the developmental approach attempts to account for changes in interaction over the family's life span.

Here again the concepts of role and position are important, but they have been invested with a longitudinal dimension, becoming "role sequences" and "positional careers" [5]. Also of importance to this approach is the concept of developmental tasks. This is a neo-Freudian conception defined by Havighurst (1948) as "a task which arises at or about a certain period in the life of an individual, successful achievement of which leads to his happiness and success with later tasks while failure leads to unhappiness within the individual, disapproval by society and difficulty with later tasks." This becomes a definition of family developmental tasks by reading "family" for "individual" above. A complication is introduced, however, by the fact that these tasks are faced simultaneously by family members who are themselves at different stages of development.

Related to these concepts is the notion of family life cycle, or family

[51] Rodgers, R. Toward a theory of family development. *Journal of Marriage and Family*, 1964, **26**, 262-270.

career. According to this concept, the family passes through several stages of development, much as the individual does. The delineation of these developmental stages has been the object of some beginning research. Duval and Hill [52], Duval [53], Feldman [50], and Rodgers [54] have all presented schemata for the analysis of the family life cycle, based primarily on demographic factors such as age of oldest child, age of youngest and oldest child, age of mother, number of years married.

From the preceding, we may conclude that families and individuals develop in different ways in response to a complex of factors, some peculiar to the family, some to the social environment. A teenager, for example, with parents who are in their fifties is essentially different from one whose parents are in their mid-thirties.

Other demographic factors also influence the successful completion of the family's developmental tasks. For example, the competent rearing of children, as viewed by the middle class at any rate, is partly contingent upon education of the parents, level of income, size of family, and many other factors.

The variables investigated by studies using the developmental approach have been numerous and far-ranging. Marital adjustment and satisfaction [50, 55-57], the effects of parenthood upon the marital

[52] Duval, E., & Hill, R. *Report of the committee on dynamics of family interaction*. Washington, D.C.: National Conference on Family Life, 1948 (mimeograph).
[53] Duval, E. *Family development*. Philadelphia: Lippincott, 1957.
[54] Rodgers, R. *Improvement in the construction and analysis of family life cycle categories*. Kalamazoo: Western Michigan University, 1962.
[55] Monahan, T. When married couples part: Statistical trends and relationships in divorce. *American Sociological Review*, 1962, 27, 240-244.
[56] Blood, R., & Wolfe, D. *Husbands and wives*. New York: Free Press of Glencoe, Inc., 1960.
[57] Bowerman, C. Adjustment in marriage: Over-all and in specific areas. *Sociology and Social Research*, 1957, 41, 257-263.

dyad [40, 58, 59], the marital dyad after children have left the home [50, 60-62] are only a sampling of the many variables that have been considered by develpmental studies to date.

A serious difficulty inherent in the developmental approach is presented by, ironically enough, its primary focus upon the family through time. There are practical difficulties involved in following the same group of families over their entire life cycles. Several alternative strategies have been proposed to obviate this difficulty—a synthetic pattern of development created from cross-sectional data, retrospective history-taking within families, segmented longitudinal designs, that is, following the same families through a shorter period of time. Hill and Rodgers [63], in a review of research employing a developmental approach, describe a study by Feldman [50], in which he used segmented longitudinal panels with controls to capture families in transition from one stage of the life cycle to the next.

Begun in 1958, the study was based on data gathered from a sample of 852 couples living in an upper-middle-class urban setting in upstate New York. The sample provided a cross-section from early marriage to old age in an attempt to highlight the transitions accomplished in the entire family career. Periods of greatest change were used as reference points for more intensive, short-term longitudinal studies of the families. The cross-sectional approach has the major advantage of being

[58] LeMasters, E. Parenthood as crisis. *Marriage and family living*, 1957, **19**, 352-355.

[59] Feldman, H. *The development of the husband-wife relationship: A Report of Research.* Ithaca, N.Y.: Cornell University, 1965.

[60] Axelson, L. Personal adjustment in the postparental period. *Marriage and Family Living*, 1960, **22**, 66-68.

[61] Sussman, M. Activity patterns of postparental couples and their relationship to family continuity. *Marriage and Family Living*, 1955, **17**, 338-341.

[62] Deutscher, I. *Married life in the middle years*, Kansas City, Mo.: Community Studies, 1959.

[63] Hill, R., & Rodgers, R. The developmental approach. In Harold T. Christensen (Ed.) *Handbook of Marriage and the Family*. Chicago: Rand McNally & Co., 1964.

more feasible and subject to wider application through the use of sampling techniques. The shorter longitudinal panels help to describe in depth significant events in the family career by studying families before and after their occurrence. Those families from the original sample who for some reason do not accomplish the transition are then available to serve as controls.

During the initial cross-sectional phase, a cycle consisting of eleven stages was developed, permitting the investigator to sort out the effects of such factors as length of marriage, the birth of the first child and subsequent children, the influence of level of education, religious affiliation, and others upon the husband-wife relationship. The nature of this relationship was indexed by several variables: patterns of communication and the extent to which communication had integrative or disintegrative consequences; marital satisfaction over the life cycle; the locus of marital authority; and mode of response to marital conflict.

The full design calls for the careful sampling of categories representing all the stages of family development through a two-phase system of interviews. The first phase attempts to capture information characteristic of the marital dyad in the stage of development in which they are presently located. The second phase is designed to be carried out late enough so that a significant number of couples would have passed on to the next developmental stage. Those couples who failed to make the transition would serve as controls for comparison with the others.

Using this kind of attack, it is possible to focus on the periods of family development where stress is greatest—from childless companions to new parents, from preschool children to school-age children, from teenagers in the home to empty nest. Each of these offers the possibility for dramatic changes in role content and positions. By sampling at strategic times, it should be possible to observe enough families accomplishing the transition to provide a wealth of data.

Many of the distinguishing characteristics of the developmental conceptual approach seem to have the potential for integrating some of the previously described frameworks, since its major concerns overlap several concept areas. It takes note, for example, that the quality and quantity of interactions among family members varies with the developmental level of the family. For example, data from the Feldman study described above reveal that level of satisfaction is equally high for newly-married and aged couples, yet an analysis shows that the components of satisfaction vary markedly. As progress is made through the life cycle, the salience of other social institutions for the family varies also. The school, government, the church, and the economic institution all vary in importance with changes in family stage.

The developmental approach offers several important relationships to Leighton's hypothesis:

(1) There are certain individual and family developmental tasks which must be accomplished in order to complete succeeding developmental tasks.

(2) The family as a system is affected by its relationship to other social systems requiring different kinds of transactions at different stages of family development.

(3) An integrated society is one which provides mechanisms for facilitating the accomplishment of socially prescribed developmental tasks.

The developmental approach would evaluate the effectiveness of the family in terms of its capacity of accomplishing developmental tasks, and its ability to relate effectively with other social systems. The designs propagated by this approach seem particularly applicable to the testing of the Leighton hypothesis. While the gross effects of community disintegration upon the prevalence of psychiatric disorder have to some extent been identified and described [64, 65], adequate

[64] Leighton, A. *My name is legion.* New York: Basic Books, Inc., 1959.
[65] Srole, L. *et al. Mental Health in the Metropolis.* Vol. I: the Midtown Manhattan Study. New York: McGraw-Hill Book Co., Inc., 1962.

research methods must be devised for investigating individual variation in the experiencing of social processes, so that the significance for mental health emerges.

Using the techniques devised by developmental researchers, the stages during which mental health problems appear could be highlighted. Cross-comparisons between families in integrated and disintegrated communities, or between families displaying psychiatric problems and healthy families within communities, taking advantage of longitudinal aspects of developmental research, should reveal transitional factors which bear upon the problem. Moreover, the developmental framework admits the use of variables which other frameworks would be unable to accomodate. In a problem as complex as that presented by Leighton's hypothesis, this flexibility makes it an approach of inestimable value.

SUMMARY

The foregoing treatment of the various conceptual frameworks employed in the study of the family should make it clear that there is wide overlap between them. The major themes of sociology and psychology run through all of them, and any attempt to classify all studies of the family would result in a taxonomical farce.

Perhaps it would be more helpful to think of these approaches not as discrete explanatory models, but as providing different perspectives of the same phenomena. Man has recently gained the ability to create social problems of a magnitude never before anticipated. Leighton's hypothesis concerning the inability of some to withstand the pressures of society is only one among many which eventually will have to be solved. Solutions will not be forthcoming if every problem is viewed from only one perspective.

9

Blue-Collar Marriage

MIRRA KOMAROVSKY, Ph.D.

A familiar refrain runs through the writings on the American family: "This is a study of a middle-class and a college-educated segment of the population." In recent years, the civil rights movement and the War on Poverty have drawn unprecedented attention to the poor—the deprived ethnic and racial minorities and the unemployed in depressed areas. Yet the socio-economic stratum in between has been relatively neglected in sociological studies. I refer to stable, employed manual or blue-collar wage-earners who are free of the disadvantages of racial and ethnic minorities and function pretty much unaided by existing welfare programs. The present study of fifty-eight blue-collar marriages was undertaken to help fill this gap in our knowledge, a gap which is, moreover, greater with regard to marriage than to child-rearing practices and parent-child relationships [1]. The present study sought to correct still another imbalance. Family studies have in the past depended predominantly upon reports of the wives. We, on the other hand, have interviewed the husbands as well.

From a theoretical point of view one of the major purposes of the study was to ascertain whether a number of well-known generalizations about marriage, derived from the studies of college-educated respond-

[1] Komarovsky, M., *Blue-collar marriage.* New York: Random House, Inc., 1964, Vintage Paperback, Random House, Inc., 1967.

ents, constitute true universals for our society or turn out to be class-linked. Another theoretical concern was with the distinction between cultural values and norms, on the one hand, and actual behavior on the other, and the congruences and discrepancies between the ideal and the actual. If behavior departs from the norm, what accounts for the discrepancy and what consequences does it have for family relationships?

The initial decision was to study a homogeneous group and to select white, Protestant couples, under 40 years of age, with at least one child, schooling not higher than high school, and the husbands presently employed in manual (largely semiskilled) jobs. The actual sample corresponded to these specifications with few exceptions of mixed religious marriages.

The major source of the respondents came from the city directory of a community (with some 50,000 inhabitants) we have named Glenton. Although practical difficulties prohibited the use of a random sample, there is no reason to suspect that the group included an overrepresentation of problem families.

The minimum number of hours spent with each family was six, including two interviews of two hours each with the wife and one two-hour interview with the husband. Some persons were seen four or five times and several additional joint interviews were conducted with husband and wife.

SUBSTANTIVE FINDINGS

Of the numerous facets of marriage covered in the study, such as division of labor, sexual and power relationships, ties with kin, leisure time activities, and others, this paper will select the patterns of marital communication and, more specifically, those involving psychic intimacy, self-disclosure, or emotional sharing. The normative expectations with regard to such sharing were ascertained by means of several "projective" test stories as well as by direct questions. The actual patterns of communication were the subject of quite elaborate scrutiny. The emotional concens of each were studied through a systematic inventory of areas of life—such as homemaking, the provider's job, children, relatives, recreation, and the like. Each respondent was asked to describe situations in a given area which, in the week or two proceeding the interview and also in general, stimulated feelings of pleasure and stress. Having ascertained those events, the respondent was asked with whom, if at all, was a particular experience discussed.

The results will be presented first for the group as a whole. If it is one of the functions of modern marriage to share one's hurts, worries, and hopes with another person, almost one-third of these working men and their wives fail to find such fulfillment. Moreover, the breaks in the marriage dialogue are not a matter of preference. They result from abortive attempts at communication, frustrated by what is felt to be the mate's lack of interest or an unsatisfactory response. On the other hand, almost one-half of the respondents do share their feelings fully or even very fully with their mates. The intermediate group falls into the category of "moderate" self-disclosure.

But these general findings obscure some consistent differences within our sample. Despite the initial intention to select a homogeneous group, the findings revealed striking differences both in normative expectations and in actual patterns of communication between the high school graduates, on the one hand, and those with less than high school education, on the other. These differences are not necessarily attributable solely to formal schooling. There is evidence to indicate that the high school graduates in our group have come from more affluent families with somewhat higher socio-economic background than was true of the less educated. Whatever the explanation, the high school graduates tend to endorse the middle-class values as to companionship and emotional sharing in marriage. Thus, a 27-year-old high school graduate, a truck driver, when asked whether women in his opinion had more need of heart-to-heart talk than men, said, "They both need each other. That's one of the purposes of marriage." To the question, "What helps you to overcome bad moods?" his answer was, "To talk about it with my wife." They made it a point, he said, when they were first married that if something was wrong, they would speak out. If her behavior puzzles him, "I make her clarify it . . . what goes on between my wife and I stays with us. I never talk to anyone about it. I am supposed to be adult; that is part of adult life." Again, a 33-year-old bottler in a beer company testified: "I can't think of anything my wife and I wouldn't tell each other that we'd tell someone else. I suppose there are some things one doesn't want to be thinking even, and so a husband wouldn't want to talk about it. But anything a husband can talk about, he can talk about to his wife, *at least I think he should* [italics ours]. And a 27-year-old high school graduate, the wife of a machinist commented: "If a wife can't talk to her husband [about very personal things], she can't talk to anyone."

Not only are such views not expressed in other interviews, but indeed different attitudes are explicitly stated. For example, asked whether she thought it was in general difficult for a husband to understand his wife, a 28-year-old woman with eight years of schooling, said, "Well, men and women are different. They each go their separate ways. A man does his work and a woman does her work and how can they know what it's all about?" When, after a long series of questions on communication, the interviewer remarked that the wife appeared to talk more easily to her girl friend and to her sister than to her husband, she exclaimed, "But they are girls!" A 21-year-old wife (with ten years of schooling) remarked, "Men are different, they don't feel the same as us. That's the reason men are friends with men, and women have women friends."

For the less educated the principal ties of marriage were seen as sexual union, complementary tasks, and mutual devotion. As to friendship, each spouse was expected to turn to members of his or her own sex.

The findings about actual communication parallel those concerning normative expectations. The high school graduates, both male and female, share their experiences in marriage much more fully than do the less educated persons. Sixty-five percent of the former, but only 36 percent of the less educated, rate our grades of "full" or "very full" disclosure. At the other extreme, "meager" or "very meager" communication characterize only 12 percent of high school graduates but as many as 41 percent of the less educated. The difference between the two educational groups persists when the comparison is controlled for the duration of marriage.

A threat to the validity of these ratings derives from variations in the educational level of respondents. People with low verbal skills may talk less in general: a larger segment of their communication may be nonverbal. As a safeguard, the grade of "meager" disclosure was never given merely because there was little conversation. It required positive evidence that some significant experiences were withheld from the mate. Additional proof was frequently furnished by the fact that these particular experiences were shared with others.

The high school spouses not only communicate more fully, but use each other more frequently as aid in periods of stress. In answer to our question: "What helps you in bad moods" our respondents listed a variety of aids, both solitary activities and relationships with others. The spouse as a source of such aid was mentioned more frequently by both husbands and wives among the high school graduates than was the case among the less educated.

The meager marital communication may have, incidentally, a special significance for the older men because fewer of them have confidants outside the home. The grandmother continues to perform functions in the lives of her married children, whereas a working-class grandfather is not similarly involved. Lack of close ties with co-workers on the job or with friends, the absence of joint social life with couples or of club membership—all result in a high degree of social isolation for many of the older men.

The differing values with regard to marriage held by the two educational groups no doubt play a part in their actual patterns of communication. But this is not the complete explanation. We have discerned a number of socially structured barriers to communication, those rooted in conditions of life and in certain by-products of a shared culture, and many of these barriers appear to be especially character-istic of the less educated respondents. We refer to the sharp differentiation in the interests of the sexes so that neither can serve as satisfactory audience for the mate, to the strict division of labor within the home, to the expectation that home and work should be kept separate, to the general impoverishment of life.

One of the major barriers to communication derives from what we have termed the "trained incapacity to share," typical especially of the less educated husbands. The ideal of masculinity into which they were socialized inhibits expressiveness both directly, with its emphasis on reserve, and indirectly, by identifying personal interchange with the feminine role. Childhood and adolescence spent in an environment in which feelings were not named, discussed, or explained strengthened these inhibitions. In adulthood they extend beyond culturally demanded reticence—the inhibitions are now experienced not only as "I shouldn't," but as "I cannot." In explaining instances of reserve in marriage many more husbands than wives say: "It is hard to talk about such things."

The strength of such norms is demonstrated in the section of the interview dealing with feelings of anger and hurt. Men and women admit the experience of anger with nearly identical frequency but twice as many women as men admitted having hurt feelings occasionally. This sex difference could hardly be attributed to the greater sensitivity of females in general. Such an explanation fails because among the high school graduates the sex difference narrows: 88 percent of the women and 83 percent of the men admit occasional feelings of hurt. The high school husband may have a less rigid norm of masculinity that allows him to admit hurt and even to ask for solace more readily than is true of the less educated men.

A major effort of the study was directed toward tracing the consequences of these patterns of communication for coping with marital conflict and for marital happiness. The relationship between communication and happiness is complex and space does not permit full discussion. Stated briefly, despite their higher expectations, the high school graduates, on the average, expressed more satisfaction with their marriages, although, of course, happy marriages were enjoyed also by many of the less educated couples.

THEORETICAL IMPLICATIONS

So much for some of our findings. I should like to turn to certain theoretical issues raised by them.

The theory that illuminates Glenton's marital problems bears little resemblance to the prevalent theories of social problems. In contemporary writings, social pathology is generally associated with anomie or breakdown of social norms and with normative ambiguities and conflicts. But Glenton's families are stable and respectable and enjoy a high degree of moral concensus. They share deeply internalized and common values. There is remarkably little disagreement about task allocation, marital roles, or child-bearing values. The consensus embraces also the parental families. The gap between generations is relatively narrow. The young mothers, for example, have not discovered Dr. Spock; they turn to their mothers as guides. The same small circle of relatives and very few friends serves as the reference group in all areas of life. The isolation from many institutions of the larger society contributes to cultural cohesion and minimizes institutional conflicts.

Despite this cultural integration, symptoms of social disorganization abound. The family is disorganized in the sense that "collective purposes and individual objectives of its members are less fully realized than they could be in an alternative workable system" [2]. A high proportion of Glenton's husbands and wives (about one-third) expressed serious dissatisfaction with their marriages, the wives being particularly dissatisfied with marital communication. Withdrawal, interspersed with violent quarreling or drinking, are not productive techniques for coping with marital conflicts, and we have occasionally been able to trace their cumulative result in a serious breakdown of marital interaction. Inability to find emotional relief within marriage builds up tension with unfavorable consequences for child-rearing or the performance of the provider on the job.

It may be readily admitted that Glenton does not exhibit any widespread adultery, illigitimacy, juvenile delinquency, or desertion. But even if we grant that such extreme forms of social deviation do tend to be associated with moral dissensus and anomie, we must guard against a certain overemphasis. If social ills are frequently the product of moral confusion, it does not necessary follow that clear moral directives and consensus are synonymous with mental or social health. Values may be internalized and shared and yet be dysfunctional under given conditions. In Glenton, it is not the failure to maintain traditional social patterns but the failure to modify them that accounts for some marital problems; in a period of rapid change, effective socialization into traditional patterns may contribute to social disorganization.

The sharp differentiation of masculine and feminine roles and the absence of the expectation of friendship in marriage are cases in point. Even when fully accepted by both partners these cultural patterns create difficulties for each. The husband pays a price for his relative exemption from domestic duties. Irritability, apathy, desire for a job outside the home—these are the reactions of some women to the domestic routine unrelieved by companionship with their husbands.

[2] Merton, R. K., & Nisbet, R. A., (Eds.), *Contemporary social problems,* New York: Harcourt, Brace Co., 1961, p. 720.

One husband baffled by his wife's frequent depressions consulted a relative who told him that women are subject to fits of "neurasthenia." He could not perceive any connection between his neglect of his wife and her condition because he behaved in what was, for his group, the accepted way. Some situations create frustrations even when they do not violate any norms. The young wife who has no expectation of friendship in marriage can still feel lonely. The young husband who never expected a wife to share his interests can still experience boredom with her conversation.

A marriage institutionalized on the basis of sharp segregation of sex roles and a certain reserve in marital interaction can and has functioned in many societies. But it requires certain supports, such as the availability of relatives and same-sex friends. But geographical mobility of Western societies tends to separate married couples from kin and trusted friends. The emotional support and other functions performed by these primary groups are no longer operative. These older forms of marriage may become increasingly unsuitable if the following prediction by a government agency proves accurate: "Many more of our workers than in the past must have, or develop, the mobility to shift jobs . . . Many may have to change their residence as well as their occupation" [3].

Another example of dysfunctional values and norms is the rigid ideal of masculinity with its consequence of the "trained incapacity to share." But the survival of dysfunctional patterns is not the only source of social disorganization in Glenton. The others, however, again do not involve moral dissensus or anomie. For example, for all their isolation from the mainstreams of our society, Glenton's couples have been stimulated to aspire to certain economic and noneconomic goals which they have difficulty in attaining for a variety of socially structured reasons. This discrepancy between aspirations and reality causes strain,

[3] Department of Labor release published in *The New York Times,* September 20, 1963.

but it does not lead to the rejection of legitimate means for the attainment of goals. The families are not sufficiently alienated from the dominant social order to countenance crime or deviation. Were the Glenton residents themselves asked to rank their difficulties, the economic situation would head the list. For the man, the economic difficulties have a special emotional significance—they undermine his self-esteem. For example, he is concerned about parental responsibilities. Our question, "Would you like your son to follow in your line of work?" was generally answered negatively. "No, I would like him to do a lot better." At the same time the fathers had doubts about their ability to provide their children with the necessary means of advancement. Their relatively low occupational and educational resources create a wide-gulf between desired goals and attainments. But we illustrate a similar strain in a noneconomic sphere. The high school graduates, as we have indicated, were on the average more happily married than the less educated couples. But there were some among the former, who, having been exposed to the newer values of marital companionship, found it, nevertheless, difficult to realize them in practice. These couples knew that husbands and wives were supposed to talk with one another but they had little to say. The impoverishment of life and the segregation in the interests of the sexes contributed to this paucity of communication. The acceptance of the new values of companionship made some high school couples feel all the more inadequate.

The reference to family disorganization raises a methodological problem long recognized in cross-national research but applying especially to the study of class differences within our own society. The ever present danger in comparative studies, all the greater when the cultural differences are subtle, is that the cues upon which the observer has always depended to assess behavior will mislead him or that he will project upon his respondents the emotions he himself would experience in given situations. Might our diagnosis of family disorganization in

Glenton merely reflect the reaction of the middle-class observer to a style of marriage which offends his sensibilities? It must be granted that for all the dissatisfaction expressed by Glenton husbands and wives, the families continue to function without any social aids or controls. But if disorganization was not extreme enough to require social intervention, it existed nonetheless. We have demonstrated that these personal dissatisfactions tended to have deleterious consequences for child-rearing, home-making, adjustment of the provider on the job, and other family functions. Moreover, the nuclear family is increasingly expected to provide the emotional support or "tension-management" no longer supplied to the same extent by the extended family or the neighborhood. This being the case, marital unhappiness by definition implies the failure of this social system to attain one of its goals.

To turn to another example, does the inarticulateness of the less educated husband, his lack of introspection, his inability to express hurt, his social isolation in later years—all add up to psychopathology, or do these merely represent a style of life unappealing to the gregarious middle-class American? The blue-collar worker himself, surrounded as he is by others sharing the same patterns, may just possibly be well adjusted to his state.

The Glenton study did not use any personality tests and made no attempt to assess individual mental health. But the relationship between social isolation and mental health is attracting increasing attention. Studies that measure only the frequency (as against intimacy) of social contacts report a modest association between social isolation and psychological maladjustment. But at least in one study of the aged, which included the *quality* of social ties, a positive relationship was found between the existence of a confidant and indicators of psychological adjustment [4].

[4] Lowenthal, M. F., & Haven, C., Interaction and adaptation: Intimacy as a critical variable, *American Sociological Review*, February, 1968, *33*, (1).
See also, Jourard, S. M., Self-disclosure and other cathexis, *Journal of Abnormal and Social Psychology*, 1959, *59*, 428-431.

Whatever the facts in this particular case, the issue was raised in order to emphasize the need for added rigor in diagnosing personal and social disorganization in comparative studies.

To conclude, the central theoretical interest of the study may lie in its portrayal of a stable, morally homogeneous group of families which, despite this consensus, suffers from many strains. Given the almost exclusive current emphasis on anomie and dissensus as the root of social problems, the study may thus provide a useful correction.

10

Job-cultures and Mental Health

BERTON H. KAPLAN, Ph.D.

Contributors

Isidor Chein, Ph.D.	Alexander H. Leighton, M.D.
Nicholas Freydberg, Ph.D.	Dorothea C. Leighton, M.D.
Lawrence Hinkle, M.D.	Stanley T. Michael, M.D.
Raymond Illsley, Ph.D.	Jane M. Murphy, Ph.D.
Thomas Langner, Ph.D.	William F. Whyte, Ph.D.

INTRODUCTION [1]

This Seminar focused on the individual's view of his environment, as distinguished from processes existing in the social unit. This focus narrowed to one of the systems in this environment, the work situation, and two work places where relevant research was available were dealt with at length, the automotive assembly line and the circumstances of incentive pay in a skilled task setting.

The automotive assembly line appears to be a coercive place where the moving conveyor belt imposes severe restrictions on physical movement and opportunity for social interaction. Minimal skills are

[1] The summary was originally prepared by Nicholas Freydberg, Ph.D.

required and there is little reason for acquiring more proficiency to do the simple, monotonous tasks. Chances to improve one's lot are remote as relatively few worth-while jobs are available off the line, and so unskilled workers have little hope of bettering themselves outside the plant. The assembly line worker's future even on the line faces the threat of diminishing ability to withstand the exhausting physical demands made upon him by the pace of the unending moving belt.

The Seminar discussion here took two directions. In one, an attempt was made to distinguish the dimensions in this specific work place that might be generalized to other work situations. A number of these were suggested as possibly falling under the rubric of the parent-child nurturance relationship (the desire to be taken care of) as, for example, recognition, admiration, supervision, security, the physical conditions of work, etc. Another category might be the number of options available in such areas as social interaction, task variability, etc.

The other direction dealt with the possibilities of relationships between these dimensions and the mental health of the worker. A routine or boring task was not believed to be a sufficient reason for disturbance. In part, at least, other factors such as social interaction, autonomy, etc., might determine the degree of job satisfaction. One proposal, in fact, was that routine jobs of an automatic nature or ones at the other end that keep the mind active may be the best in this regard, while the ones in between, the dull type that at the same time demand constant attention, may be the more noxious. From another viewpoint, the opportunity to use one's skills may be rewarding, but it can be counterbalanced by the measure of responsibility borne by the worker. An illustration offered was of a tool and die maker who with almost complete autonomy on the task which might take many months generated increasing tension as he approached completion. He had good reason since a single mistake would require that he begin all over again. Job satisfaction might be reflected from such elements as "closure," the completion of a job, as contrasted with never experiencing this, which brings to mind the assembly line worker who tightens a few bolts and never is able to say of the finished product, "this is mine." Some jobs appear to have traction, the quality of involving the worker in its immediate completion, while others don't. However, the question remains open as to whether job satisfaction in its own right is correlated with mental disorder.

The second illustration of a work situation faced the mental health problem more directly. Here the men were employed on a variety of skilled tasks and each could earn incentive pay based on his own production. An understanding among the workers limited an individual to producing not more than a certain percentage above 100 percent. Eighty-four men who had been in the department for a certain period of years participated in the research. Fifty of these abided by the group norm, nine of the men exceeded it, and twenty-five consistently fell below 100 percent. Skill was not an important factor as all were experienced men, and some of the lowest producers had received a top rating by management before the installation of the incentive. It was discovered that nine of the men had an ulcer history or symptoms of incipient ulcers, and all were in the group of fifty who abided by the norm. The explanation offered by the invesitgator was that those hewing to the group norm found themselves under the cross-pressure of wanting to earn more money while at the same time desiring approval of their fellows. The over-producers elimated the pressure of the norm by refusing to accept this restriction, and they experienced no conflict, while the under-producers by refusing to accept the dollar reward similarly were not torn by the opposing forces.

These two illustrations, as well as others offered in less detail, produced some hypotheses about the dynamics related to mental disturbance in different kinds of work situations. One conjecture was that the assembly line with its frustrations associated with accomplishment, growth, recognition, etc., was in the main a reality one external to the individual and not a moral one involving guilt. The prognosis in mental health terms was the likelihood of neurasthenic symptoms such as boredom, inability to become interested, a rigid constriction in interests and activities. In contrast, the incentive pay circumstance where rewards and norms are involved would be more likely to induce symptoms associated with the kinds of anxiety related to dependency needs.

Prior to taking up the work situation, the Seminar group inspected the effect of change in interaction patterns in an adolescent gang and the addiction of some of its members to drugs. The crucial determinant may depend on the ability of the individual gang member to develop relationships outside of the group at the time that dissolution threatens its existence because of movement toward adulthood. Prior patterns of leadership or followership in the gang are not necessarily related to this ability, but rather degree of involvement in the gang and lack of capacity to make adult commitments. It was suggested that people have capacities for leadership in some situations and not in others. Possibly change in interaction patterns, rather than quantity, may have significant associations with mental health.

Some points were also made regarding the process of disintegration. The concept is being used in different ways by various participants of the Seminar, and, at times, interchangeably with disorganization. The term "environment" likewise is being employed for a variety of contexts. Some commonality of definition is indicated.

Another session of the Seminar continued its focus on the environment as the individual experiences it. For our purposes, the discussion can be grouped into three content areas: the work place, other systems or combinations of systems in the individual's total environment, and methodological problems confronting research of this type in an urban setting.

The Work Place

A previous meeting ended with dimensions of the job situation that might contribute to the worker's satisfaction or discontent; the next meeting continued this exploration. A preference among discussants toward democratic supervision as a benign influence had been evident, but research indicates that this is not necessarily so. The task situation can be the determinant. Too much supervision on a routine task can be noxious, but the exercise of close control appears to be preferred when the task is more demanding of skills and the responsibility is great. The "fit" between a worker's expectations and the judgment of his qualifications by others can determine not only the degree of satisfaction, but the significance of the work system to him as well. This matter of importance of work and, closely related to it, the extent to which it is segregated from or integrated into the individual's other interaction systems, also can be influenced by the "degrees of freedom" the worker sees in his choice of job and the opportunity he has to mold it to meet his own needs.

How important is the job in relation to other roles? For certain ethnic and socio-economic groups, it may be closely interwoven into the total social fabric of the individual, as in the case of Puerto Rican women working in the garment industry and clustered together in the same residential area. In regard to emotional disturbance, quite probably it is of less significance to them than family affairs and other group affiliations. Studies of women who work show that the importance of the job is not as great as their roles of wife and mother, and it is not as salient as it is to men. Saliency, too, is likely to vary according to class, possibly influenced by the "freedom of choice" and "fit" dimensions earlier mentioned. The job can be important in another way than saliency, for it can influence the other systems, as in the case of fishermen away at sea for extended periods, forcing their wives to take over almost all of the parental functions. In converse, marital roles can become interchangeable, as occurs with railroad workers because of the shift nature of the occupation, and when wives, too, are employed.

Research dealing with the influence of social systems on mental health, if it attempts to enter this investigation via the work place, has to deal with some serious possibilities for bias. For one, the probability of self-selection exists in certain industries and organizations, as, for example, psychopathic types in salt fishing in Aberdeen. Social factors often are influential; among telephone operators certain religious and national groups are attracted, and others repelled by the public image of the company. Of vital importance here is the factor of selectivity as it undoubtedly operates to exclude those less fit to obtain regular employment.

Other Systems in the Environment

It was suggested that an individual's "fit" in his situation in life, in terms of background, temperament, and experience, seemed to be related to manifestations of illness. A Negro boy involved in narcotics in Harlem may be evidencing less pathology than a similarly involved white boy in Riverdale. The Negro boy is moving with a social force, the white boy against it. Jahoda, in fact, proposed learning about an environmental setting by identifying those fitting best into it. But what about "fit" in an environment in flux? Perhaps, then, flexibility becomes a crucial characteristic. Among a group of uprooted Chinese, the least symptomatic were shallow in their attachments, able to live fluidly, and almost sociopaths.

This concept of "fit" and its implications for maladjustment is dramatically demonstrated in the circumstances of Puerto Rican women who have located work suitable for their skills, in contrast to failure in an equivalent "fit" by their menfolk. A recent study in Nigeria found village women less disturbed than the men. Little had changed for the women, but the men were themselves torn between the cross-pressures of "going European" or "staying native." Somewhat similar events are recorded for the American Indian. In the Stirling Study, women with education beyond high school were worse off than men with the same level of education. There was nothing for the women to do with theirs.

The issue of geographic community and nongeographic systems of interaction came to the forefront again. The latter, probably scattered across a wide territorial range, are apt to be a characteristic of urban areas such as New York City, although, certainly, the city must also contain some neighborhoods of a geographic type and gradations of both. Modern communication and improved transportation have widened the spread of interaction, and, where previously this had particular application to upper socio-economic groups, it now must apply to most of the scale. It may be that at least part of the research effort will have to be directed at an investigation of these networks, and, where the overlap of systems in such a network is minimal, it is likely to be difficult to locate a social process of disintegration. It would seem to follow that a more loosely related network would provide an individual with greater freedom of choice in his relationships, in comparison with the geographic situation where propinquity is a compelling influence. Movement from one area in New York to another would be substantially another matter than moving from one village in Nova Scotia to another, with the consequence in the latter instance of loss of whole sets of acquaintanceships.

Methodology

A number of investigators have worked on the problem of identifying the systems that comprise an individual's environment and assessing their saliency and amount of harmony or integration. Merton and Kitt's "community of interest" refers, in effect, to the location of the reference group. An idea broached during the discussion was the compiling of a matrix of interaction systems participated in by the individual, somewhat as was done by Bott in her study of intercommunication among families in London. The extent to which these overlapped in membership could be determined in this manner. If frequency of interaction also was ascertainable, it might prove to have relevance for saliency.

Homans' concept of "status congruence" deals with the notion that each of us has several statuses in the community, ethnic, sex, religion, education, etc., and the extent to which these are at equal levels determines the strain on the person. There are difficulties, however, in using subjective assessments of the saliency of roles. One investigator discovered a tendency to name someone higher as the closest friend, although interaction was infrequent. The place of interview seems to exert an influence; if it is at work, the problems there are stressed, and if at home, this area appears to be the more salient. But the most formidable methodological problem deals with the contamination of the independent and the dependent variables if one approaches an assessment of the individual's environment through his focus. An objective appraisal would be a safer procedure.

A number of researchers have found a relationship between social class and mental illness, but this appears to have added little to our understanding. A proposal was made to include some vertical as well as horizontal class variables as the determinants in the selection of the population, the specific suggestion being a job-culture combination encompassing groups like Jewish furriers, Irish policemen, etc. This combination can link class and social systems with culture, adding adhesives of sentiment and communication, and it provides the opportunity to study their congruence or conflict. It is an atmosphere in which people spend much of their lives and one in which the prevailing conditions probably can be determined. One question here is how much of New York City can you account for in this way? Perhaps an answer is that you need not confine yourself to these particular variables; three or four others might slice up New York City in sufficiently homogeneous units, and between them encompass enough of the city. Perhaps an approach through multicraft unions is a means for reaching important segments.

The place of residence, to present another view, has certain advantages. First of all, you're beginning with the primary family unit, which is likely to be more relevant to the individual's mental health than any other interaction system. It includes components that are missing in the work situation—nonworking housewives, young people, the aged, and the ill—and it is not subject to the selective bias introduced by such criteria as holding down a job. A moot point is whether these elements would be included in a job-culture or another multivariable criteria approach, which, although entering through occupation, would presumably fan out to include the complex of relationships.

SEMINAR DISCUSSION ON JOB-CULTURES AND MENTAL HEALTH

It is clear that if you want to study the mental health implications of work you have to understand the nature of job-cultures. Indeed, the whole question of job-cultures is a most important and little examined area of inquiry.

The following discussion is rich with research suggestions for the study of job-cultures and mental health.

(Focus on individual—methodology: Could we divide New York into

"job-cultures" (defining culture as shared normative values)—Jewish furriers, Irish policemen? How much would it account for?)

A. Leighton: I wonder if it would be possible to think not of a job and not of culture, but of something that might be hyphenated as job-culture, defining culture as a group of people who share the same normative values or sentiments. Then we could see how many such groups are to be found in a city. Irish policemen would make one set; Jewish furriers might be another one. These groups might at times cut a job in part. There might be two such groups that share one occupation. Would it be feasible to try to divide New York into major globules of job-culture groups? How much of New York or Aberdeen should you actually get organized into these units? How much would be left over that wouldn't fit?

(*F. I.—methodology:* Include three or four variables, make the group large enough, and it might work, e.g., college educated broken down into large occupation groups.)

Hinkle: If one is willing to exclude from his mind the concept of a community as necessarily being a geographic unit, then I think it would work very well. I think if you categorize a group of people on the basis of having had a college education and then chop this up into a number of large segments of occupations that these college-educated people might go into, you would also find a considerable congruence in the types of communities in which they lived, in the types and amount of educations their wives have.

(*F. I.—environment:* In Nigeria hardly anything had changed for village women, but men were under cross-pressures to "go European" and to "stay native." The women seemed in better mental health.)

D. Leighton: That was very clearly demonstrated, we thought, in Nigeria. Hardly anything had changed for the women in the villages. They were doing almost the same thing as women had done for generations in Nigeria. But the men were under pressures to "go European" and to "stay native." We don't have enough material to say that the women or the men complain more. We certainly don't know how many days they stayed out of work by reason of their symptoms. But in over-all terms, the women seemed to have better mental health as compared to the men and differed in this from our other studies (except for the integrated French community in Stirling County).

(F. I.—work situation: Michigan investigators found that the amount of skill required in a job was inversely related to visits to the plant medical facilities, but that the amount of supervisory responsibility was directly related to these visits.)

Freydberg: I ran across another piece of research on the relationships between physical health and work skill and various kinds of work responsibility. Investigators at Michigan attempted, in two different plants, to catalog jobs according to skill and supervisory activities according to the degree of responsibility. They found that the number of times the employees visited the dispensary or medical facilities was inversely related to the amount of skill the particular job required and yet it was directly related to the amount of supervisory responsibility. In other words, the lesser skilled visited the dispensary often, but the supervisor with greater responsibility visited the dispensary more often still.

(F. I.—methodology: Risky to get dependent and independent variables from the same source, as is true if the subjective community is used as frame of reference. Research will be better with another way of determining the environment.)

A. Leighton: I would like to go back a bit and make a point with regard to this business of letting subjective communities (to which a person belongs by his own definition) act as a frame of reference. It is a methodological point and refers to the fact that I think it's risky to get both the dependent and independent variables from the same source when you're interested in studies that relate the environment of social systems to mental health. We've all done this up to now, but I think our research will be stronger if we have some way of defining the environmental state, what the environment is, and its condition in terms that are quite independent of those that are concerned with rating the mental health status. I think we should try to avoid, in future work, correlating one subjective statement by the respondent with another subjective statement from different parts of the same questionnaire.

Illsley: Is this the problem? You trace out for a given individual a pattern of activities, interactions, and relationships that describes a community. This you feel is acceptable as a description of what his community is. But the point about which you're worried is then to ask the individual which of these is more important to him, asking him to identify one above the other, one aspect of his community above another?

A. Leighton: Yes, or getting him to define his reference group and leaving it at that—without any other information, as to what (in terms of his behavior from day to day, from year to year) his reference group actually seems to be from other sources.

(F. I.—methodology: Could the Midtown technique be applied, the objective data first evaluated, and then correlations be made between this and the subjective data?

Michael: I think if you could use the same dimension here as in the Midtown Study, part of the information could be kept aside and an evaluation made first of the objective data, and then a correlation made between the subjective and the objective information.

(*F. I.—methodology:* In Aberdeen I do it by studying everybody in the community. If Mrs. Y says she interacts with Mrs. X, I also ask Mrs. X.)

Illsley: In the study I was doing, my way of getting around this was to study everybody in the same community. If Mrs. Y says that she interacts with Mrs. X, I also want to hear from Mrs. X that she interacts with Mrs. Y, or I don't accept it.

(*F. I.—methodology:* Method mentioned by Illsley is less feasible in larger populations.)

A. Leighton: This kind of technique and checking, of course, has been possible in the small communities. It gets to be less feasible in these larger populations unless it's given some special attention.

(*F. I.—methodology:* Need when interviewing to distinguish between stated reference group and statements about interaction. A tendency existed among respondents in one study to name as closest friends someone higher in social scale although interactions were infrequent.)

Langner: I think we ought to do something in interviewing to distinguish between a stated reference group and statements about interaction. I am thinking about a study of factory workers. The investigator asked them who their closest friends were. He found it was quite a common reaction that the workers would name certain individuals, but when asked: "How often in the last year have you seen this individual?" the worker would say: "Well maybe once, or, well, we didn't see him last year at all or the year before." From further tracing through it was found that the people named as closest friends tended to be individuals who were just a bit higher in the social scale. The datum regarding who are your closest friends would be significant but it wouldn't mean what it appeared to mean on the face of it.

A. Leighton: Raymond, I wanted to ask if you could say anything more about this scheme for plotting interaction groups? Have you thought of any ways of diagramming this?

(*F. I.—methodology:* You can diagram interaction for each individual by a matrix distinguishing the total groups and identifying those in which he participates. You can also determine the degree of integration of one group with another. If frequency of interaction is also obtained, it may provide saliency.)

Illsley: I've thought of ways of diagramming it, but I haven't yet thought of ways of measuring or distinguishing saliency. This is the most difficult part. For the diagram I simply worked out a kind of matrix; along one axis I would distinguish the total number of groups with which people interacted. (This in itself is a difficult thing to do without detailed interviewing.) Down the other axis I would list the same set of groups. Then I shaded in with a particular color all those groups where the group with whom a person interacted was actually within the community. Just by looking at the different patterns, you can come away with the impression of great differences between the ones that are entirely shaded and ones that are entirely unshaded. You could find this difference of pattern even in the same family, between a husband and wife.

A. Leighton: Did you make a diagram for each individual?

Illsley: For each individual, yes. That's as far as I've gotten up to now. But then you could also begin in the matrix making some kind of mark to distinguish those places where friendship cluster A interacts with friendship cluster B and so on. You could see at a glance from this the degree of integration of one group of friends with another group of friends or acquaintances. This is a clumsy method if you apply it in any kind of large scale work, but I was only using it as a way of seeing the problem. What it doesn't do, however, is show you anything whatsoever about how important any of these particular clusters or groups are to the individual.

A. Leighton: Do you have data on frequency of interactions?

Illsley: No and that is what you'd have to get in order to rate saliency.

A. Leighton: Whenever there are the same individuals in two groups, the square gets colored, as I understand it. Is that right?

Illsley: Yes.

(*F. I.—methodology:* Bott uses "integration" to refer to the extent of communicative connections in a system. What she terms "nonintegration" is total lack of communication. Our concept requires only a pattern of communication sufficient to enable the system to function.)

A. Leighton: There's one point I think could be clarified here. From what you were telling me the other day Bott used the term "integration" to mean what I would call "interconnection." That is, if you visualize all the people of a community as so many dots projected on a piece of paper, then when she speaks of integration she means that every dot knows every other dot, has communication with every other dot? When she said nonintegration it means a lack of communication. This is a different conception of disintegration from what we've been using. Although communication of some sort is a necessary condition for integration of a community system, it doesn't have to be everybody with everybody else. It has to be a pattern of communication that enables the system to function.

(*F. I.—methodology:* If you start with individuals who share many of the same attributes or associations, the likelihood is for overlap in several areas, or in similar ones, even if they are geographically dispersed.)

Hinkle: You're still talking here about intensive studies of individuals. If each individual were utterly unique, it would not only be an almost hopeless task to accomplish, but it also wouldn't matter where you started. But chances are you're going to start with individuals who share many of the same attributes or associations, even those who are geographically dispersed. This likelihood of sharing would mean that there would be overlap in several areas. If we wished, we could, for example, study the faculty, who have a predilection to settle in a particular suburban community—e.g., Pelham—and to join into various social activities and friendship activities together. I think what you're saying implies that studies, to be meaningful, should investigate the place where they send their children to school, and maybe their voting habits. I think if you made the sample large enough and were willing to include three or four variables, it might be meaningful.

Freydberg: I would like to raise an issue about this job-culture information. I suspect that it's a rather middle-class determinant and that it may not take us quite to the blue-collar area.

(F. I.—methodology: An occupational classification is a middle-class criterion. At the top of the scale are fine gradations, but the lower 60% are lumped into skilled, semiskilled, etc. If you draw in something other than occupation, it may work, such as aspects of jobs not necessarily socio-economic. In Aberdeen one might be those that lead to breaks in continuity of living together between husbands and wives, as the salt fishermen.)

Illsley: It depends how you handle it. I would agree with your point about it being a middle-class criterion. I've often been fascinated by the way in which you get series after series of socio-economic occupational classifications. They start off at the top end of the scale with fine gradations and small groups, obviously middleclass people being able to distinguish very, very clearly one small group of occupations from another. Then you get down to about 60 percent of the population, the so-called skilled and semiskilled, and nobody can distinguish between them on an occupational basis. But I think if you draw in something other than occupation you will begin to get worthwhile classifications.

In my kind of Scottish community I couldn't use variables that you could use. There are no ethnic groupings. We've got 4 percent Catholics and no Jews. It's a very different kind of community and therefore I would have to use a very different series of variables. For example, I would take people who had kids living in the community versus those who had migratory children. I'd take aspects of jobs that are not necessarily socio-economic—the kind I mentioned this morning that lead to a break between a husband and a wife—the fishermen who goes away, the shipworker, and so on. I think one would have to bring in a whole number of variables of this kind in order to make distinctions of the kind you're indicating.

(F. I.—methodology: Warner's classification, such as education, occupation, place and type of dwelling, etc., probably will do at working-class levels. Each of these large groups breaks down into finer ones, Negro telephone operators connected with migrants from British West Indies or North Carolina; barbers into Sicilian-Italians.)

Hinkle: I think the trend of the work of Warner and others is based on such phenomena as education, occupation, place and type of dwelling, type of association, single versus married. There appear to be pretty close associations between these things in our society and in European society too.

Having worked a good deal with working groups, I'm not convinced that you can't make the same sort of classifications if you go on to working-class people, even people at the very lowest level of our society. Of course you have to be willing to communicate with these people and understand them. As I mentioned to you, even though this group of telephone operators broke down into white and Negro, they were all in the same social class. Yet among the Negroes these groups were distinguished by the two or three who were connected with the British West Indies; several who were from North Carolina and Virginia, and others who had lived in this community for two to three years, or for a couple of generations. I found even with the barbers here in our hospital, that these were normally Sicilian and roughly all of the same family. This came out when I asked them if a barber whom I knew could get a job there, and they pointed out to me that not only was he not Italian (he was French Canadian whom the other group of barbers would snub), but he was not even Sicilian-Italian (they separate these from the Neapolitans and other groups). So I think each of the larger groupings will break down into finer and finer groupings.

Illsley: This is exactly what I'm saying. When you get down to this particular group of the population (skilled manual workers, and certainly semiskilled and unskilled) at that point I think you've got to begin distinguishing these people by variables other than occupation. You'll get fine distinctions but not necessarily moving down the same occupational dimension but by bringing in other things. These other things may be far more important to this individual and to his family than occupational distinctions.

(F. I.—methodology: An alternate to the working place could be the unions—electrical workers, ladies garment workers, etc. Some cut across industries, include many occupations, and their records may provide information on job settings, geographical residential distributions, etc.)

Whyte: Up to this point, I've been thinking of making an approach through the working place rather than geographically. Another approach might be through the union, particularly in a city such as New York where you have, say, the International Brotherhood of Electrical

Workers Local #3, a tremendous organization with various plants included, ranging all the way from manufacturing to construction, small operators and big operators. The management of the Union is quite a thing, and I presume they must have records on all their members. Or one could look at the garment industry through the International Ladies Garment Workers, and at the longshoremen through their union.

I don't think I'd urge this in the abstract, but it might be worthwhile consulting with people in such a union as to what kind of records they have, what kinds of job settings their members work in, and whether they have data about the geographical distribution of their members. I'm not saying commit yourself to an approach through the union but to try in one of several unions to see what you could learn about this population and how it might be socially categorized.

(*F. I.—methodology:* Which social group you start with doesn't matter as long as it is specifiable. Selection should not be limited to lower segments, and also look at complex systems such as New York medical staff.)

Hinkle: I might suggest that it doesn't really matter which one of the social groupings one takes so long as one starts with a more or less specifiable group and begins to work out and around this. For example, you could take a group such as the recent Puerto Rican migrants and find out what jobs they have and where they live. After finding out what occupations they have and who else is in these occupations, then move out from that. Probably for a beginning it would be good to select one or two sorts of groupings and also not be limited to the lower segment of society. One also ought to look at some of the more complex systems, for example, the staff of this medical center and apply the same methods so as to see what the differences are.

(*F. I.—methodology:* How can groups be chosen without contamination of the dependent variable? Preselection in industry, in family, etc., are all related to mental illness. If you're psychotic you've gone down in the system.)

Langner: I'm still confused as to how these groups can be chosen without having them be contaminated by the dependent variable. Preselection in industries and preselection of the family unit—married, unmarried, children, no children, and so forth—all these things are part of the circular relationship to mental health or disorder. Leo Srole's idea was to take aspects of the parental status as his starting point. He thinks present social status is contaminated by the mental health variable. If you're a schizophrenic, there's no doubt, I think, but that you've gone down in the system. You've dropped out of school early because of it and you don't have skills and so you're going to have low social status.

(*F. I.—methodology:* If you want to study prevalence, you need a probability sample of a geographical area. If it's how interactions within the social environment influence health, you select units with their characteristics. They're not representative and, as yet, we do not know whether they are relevant.)

Hinkle: I think this is a question of whether you wish to study prevalence related to a larger community or whether you are interested in seeing if you can find out something about mental illness. If you want to study prevalence, the thing to do is to get a probability sample of the geographic area. In New York this would be available through the census. But I think that if you are concerned with how interactions within the social environment influence health, then you have to watch some interaction processes as they go on. That means that you have to select units with all of their characteristics, and you have to understand that no one of these is in any way representative or unbiased as far as the community as a whole is concerned.

Nor would I believe at this stage of the game that you could say this type of unit is going to be more relevant, important, or enlightening than that type.

(*F. I.—methodology:* There are mental health differences relating to class which are not understood. In addition to horizontal (class) lines there are vertical ones. Job-culture may link class and social systems, with culture adding the adhesives of sentiments and communication, providing the opportunity to study their congruence or contact.)

A. Leighton: I want to say something about the class concept. It seems to me that Warner, Srole, and Hollingshead and others have done a tremendous job for the understanding of society in the emphasis they have given to social class. In looking forward and building on the work that's been done, I think it would be profitable to give less stress to the class stratification. We know that there are these mental health differences that relate to stratification, but we don't know very much about why they exist. We don't understand why everybody at the lowest level is not affected adversely. We don't know why everybody at the upper level is not healthy. In Warner's early "Yankee City Series" studies, it was apparent (as it was also to us in the studies of Bristol), that in addition to these horizontal lines there are verticals that overlap. The stratification of society is something like a stone wall. If you look at a loosely built stone wall, you can see horizontal lines there, but you also see stones that stick out through several layers, and you see that the horizontal lines are interrupted by vertical lines, and that there are lumps and chunks in the wall. We've been concentrating very heavily on the horizontal lines. It would seem that one of the things we can do with some promise of breaking new ground is to take off from that emphasis and begin to ask what units are there within a given stratum and what units are there that may cut across several of them.

There's another thing about most of the literature on class. It's fairly static in quality, and what we're concerned with is the social system.

The notion of the job-culture that came up this morning—it seems to me that with it you could link what we know about class structure and what we know about social systems. The job component of it is certainly part of the machinery that makes the community go. The cultural component not only involves the idea of interconnection, communication, and adhesion, but also congruence of norms, which is one of the things Dr. Chein brought up in the first meeting. The culture idea involves the sentiment systems and how these may be cohesive within one unit and different in another unit. Between units the sentiments and norms may be congruent or complemental or they may get into each other's way.

Freydberg: I think you can find a job-culture group that contains a large range of the social classes and yet still is organized as a work place—the hospital here is such an example.

Illsley: I think what you're saying, Alex, is that we need to move away from the kind of rather mechanical methods of social classification that have been particularly used for studies of prevalence and incidence of disease. They've been instrumental in providing gradients and hierarchies; but they've not taken us very far in the understanding of social process within the area that we're looking at.

Murphy: Do you think that the job-culture idea would provide us with a way of looking at a sufficient range of work places and situations? For example, would the assembly line group that we discussed last time have anything similar to a culture in the same sense as the Irish policemen and the Jewish furriers? Were they more mixed?

Whyte: On the particular example of the automotive assembly line, I don't know that you have any such thing right within New York City. There's a Ford assembly plant in nearby New Jersey. Plants of this nature do not tend to settle in a city of this sort.

Freydberg: But assuming that they did, you'd still have to take more than just the assembly line. You'd have to take the whole range of jobs in the plant from the highest executive to the lowest so that you would be following through or eliminating the class bias that might occur there.

Murphy: I agree. To study job situations as a system, it would seem to me, you'd have to cover all levels, and this would give you a lot of diversity.

Whyte: I haven't studied this myself but I gather you wouldn't get a great range in the assembly line plant. The jobs are engineered from some place else, and you have quite a small supervisory or management organization and this tremendous class of jobs at the bottom. If you're looking for a work situation with great diversity to make comparisons among various groups, then an assembly line wouldn't be a very good choice. You would pick the assembly line plant because you wanted to look at something regarding the pressures of this particular type of work situation.

(F. I.—methodology: Whether you pick up the collection of individuals living in proximity or working in proximity, you have to pursue each through other interaction patterns if you want to find why they stay healthy or get sick.)

Chein: It seems to me we're getting an awful lot of things confused here. One question is where do you get your base population? It seems to me, everything we have been saying is that regardless of how you define that base population, if you want to pursue the relevant social interactions of the individuals in that base population, you're going to have to pursue these individuals through social groupings that don't respect the definition of the base population. If you start with a collection of individuals living in physical proximity, or working in physical proximity, and then for some reason you want to investigate why they stay healthy or get sick (and this on the assumption that interacting with people makes a difference) then you'll have to break up those proximity patterns. You'll have to pursue the individual picked up in the factory or the one picked up in the residential neighborhood through various other kinds of interaction patterns.

In some sense we have been trying to decide the most strategic base population to start with. What we haven't indicated yet is that if we want to pursue these patterns of interaction, we pick up people on any definition and pursue them to where they lead us.

(*F. I.—methodology:* You will find some individuals whose direct interaction with others are not contingent on physical proximity, and some where it is. Some interact with the same individuals across a wide variety of situations, and for others the same ones do not persist.)

The second level of confusion seems to me to concern the implications of the properties of the association or universe of the individual. We recognize, for instance, that in some strata of whatever population is selected, we're going to find some sets of individuals whose direct interactions with other individuals are not contingent on physical proximities, and we may find other sets of individuals whose interactions with other individuals are contingent on physical proximity. You will find some sets of individuals for whom the direct interaction groups persist across a wide variety of behavioral situations, and possibly others for whom they do not persist across a wide variety of behavioral situations.

(Our problem is not to classify social groupings but to start looking at why the dimensions we are discussing may be relevant to mental health.)

Now, the confusion that I see here stems from the fact that we're assuming that this kind of a network is relevant to mental health. Why should it make a difference whether the interactional sets persist or do not persist, or whether they depend on physical proximity or do not depend on physical proximity? I think these are relevant dimensions, but I think unless we start looking at why they are relevant dimensions, we just go off into questions of how you can classify social groupings. This isn't our interest. We want to classify them in a way that's relevant to the mental health of individuals.

Now, for instance, let me take one of these. If you selected a grouping of individuals on the basis of residential proximity, or if you selected them on the basis of work proximity, and it turns out that there's a great deal of independence between the direct interaction groups and the physical proximity groups, then it seems to me there are two implications. One is that the individual in the physical location (again whether it's residential or on the job) is surrounded by individuals who are not interacting with one another and who consequently do not develop a normative structure. The person, physically, would be in a situation which is normless. (I'm taking an extreme.) To locate the normative structure of this individual is not only a job for us, but it's a job for this individual himself because it's not the pattern in his area for people to interact directly with one another. He's going to be an isolated individual unless he does find his own way of establishing connections with individuals. So he's got a task in front of him, a task which is generated by the nature of the environmental situation in which he finds himself.

Let me illustrate. I recall I once had a semester's job teaching at Brooklyn College, and I quickly discovered that nobody talked to each other in the whole psychology department. Everybody went his own way, nobody had any connection with anybody else. Simply because I had a need in this situation, I would stop when it came lunch time and I would drop in on somebody and say: "Are you going to lunch?" "Well," he said, "o.k." So I said: "How about asking so and so?" and before that semester was over, we would have 30 people going out for lunch together. This was absolutely standard. Nobody went to lunch without asking everybody else, and everybody was busy making sure that so and so had been asked.

In effect, out of my needs a social structure emerged which was different from the social structure that had existed. Interestingly enough, I was told, within a few months after I left, everybody was going to lunch by himself, and nobody was talking to one another any more. It wasn't because they resented one another, but they were being pulled in different directions. Being confronted with a situation such as that poses a problem for the individual who gets into the situation.

If we start looking at these patterns in terms of the kinds of problems that they're likely to generate for individuals, then we get the clues as to why we want to follow things up. You can look at the persistence of the interaction group across different behavioral situations. This can be good in some situations, but it can also be catastrophic as in the case where you have the boss and his mistress working in the same office. This becomes a source of strain because the imperatives associated with the two roles involved in the relationship of these people are quite different, and they're inconsistent with one another, and everybody else in this office is going to get mixed up if these are important people in the office.

On the other hand, the ability to keep on interacting with the same individuals in different behavioral settings may simplify the world for the individual. He has fewer people to adjust to, but he may also have more complex role relationships to adjust to. So it seems to me, if we simply start seeing how many different ways we can classify social relationships without pausing to say to ourselves "so what?", we are going to get awfully mixed up.

Langner: The assumption though is that we know, after twenty to thirty years of studies such as this, which types of situations to sample. When you started the discussion of everybody's going to lunch together, I thought of my daughter. She is in school where if you're not in with the group, God help you. Even the teachers get on your back. But she's very circumspect about getting into the group, and I'm sure she doesn't actually want to be part of it. So it seems that integration into the social group is what you just have to do from nursery school on up. But the business of association itself can be a positive or a negative factor, toward either extreme. So maybe you would want to select some populations that are isolated and some that are over-integrated.

Chein: I still have a bias for selecting them on a neighborhood basis but this is another theme.

(F. I.—methodology: Few neighborhoods are communities in New York. The job occupies a few hours and much depends on the rest of the day. But the job-culture unit offers an atmosphere in which people spend much of their lives. We can determine the prevailing conditions and effects here.)

A. Leighton: I would like to express a little more about what my notion was in talking about these job-cultures. I've been trying to think of some way of carving up the city into units such that people who are in those units spend most of their lives in that atmosphere and associating with other people in that unit. The limitation on the job classification alone is that people only spend the work hours there and an awful lot of their ability to stand the working hours depends on what's happening the rest of the time. The difficulty with a neighborhood study in a city is that only some people have their associations in the neighborhood. There are only some neighborhoods that are communities in the city.

This job-culture idea seemed to me to define units in which people spent most of their time and where they were bound to find a common set of values, and in which they know face-to-face many people in the network. If we find units such as the police force and the furriers, then we can begin to ask ourselves: "What are the prevailing conditions of an interaction with these?" Then we can begin to think of some scale of noxious and benign forces relevant to mental health. We'll have a unit that can be examined in these mental health terms—whether you're living among people who get in your way when you try to do something or whether you've got an anomic type of unit so you don't know what you want to do anyhow.

(*F. I.—methodology:* I prefer to start with the residential neighborhood because you're beginning with the primary family unit. My assumption is that it is more relevant to the individual's mental health than job interactions in most cases.)

Chein: Except if you start in the job situation, you'll have to pursue the individuals, among other places, into their primary family unit. One reason I prefer to start with the residential neighborhood is that you're beginning with the primary family units in the first place. Here I have a bias. My assumption is that somehow the primary family unit is more relevant to the mental health of the individual than job interactions though not in all cases and not by all means.

Hinkle: I think the problem of mental health revolves around the question of generalization within a social system. It seems to me perfectly clear that the final determinants of my health are all of those peculiar things, idiosyncratic to me—it includes not only the genetic factor but the physical atmosphere, and also my particular set of relationships with other people. I agree with that, but it is the approach of the clinician and the pathologist. I think we want to ask questions about processes that are general to a social system.

If this is a study of social psychiatry, it is a study of factors relevant to the social environment as such, that is social processes and social groupings. We are then asking ourselves what is most likely to be the most profitable social grouping to use as an approach in the city? We know that the nature of New York City is such that if we take a slice of it, such as the East Side of Manhattan, that it's just like cutting through a beehive with a butcher knife. We get all sorts of samples.

If we start with a social grouping, built around occupational as well as ethnic and social factors, then we suspect we will be able to detect irregularities to a finer degree than had previously been detected with this broader sampling by ethnic group as a whole, or by social class as a whole. I think that we have to decide right away whether this is a study of individuals at an individual clinical level or whether this is a study of social processes and social groupings in relation to mental health because I think the methods to be used would be completely different.

Whyte: I think you ought to take a position somewhere in between. In this way you could start from the occupational base, but ask yourselves: Of the occupations that you might select for a study in New York City, are there some that are more geographically based than others? I think it's very doubtful if you'd find a given workshop where everybody lives right around there. I think you might find some concentration in certain areas of people, say, in the garment trade.

A. Leighton: I don't think we can conceive of making a study of mental health without considering the family as one of the central units. I was thinking of the Irish policeman in New York and his family, which is what you can embrace in this type of job-culture concept. Whereas if you take the work place alone, the family is left out of it. Perhaps the logic of this discussion is to move on in our next meeting to taking up the family, which is the third item on the latest agenda.

(F. I.—methodology: If we take the job situation we're mainly dealing with men and missing components of the population bound to the residential neighborhoods—youth, housewives, the aged, etc.)

Chein: May I make a point about the strategic implications of residential neighborhoods versus job? I think a major consideration is the population problem. If we take the job situation, we're mainly interested in the male population. Women work, of course, but they are much less likely to be centrally involved in their work than the men. Also in the work situation, we're missing components of the population that are relatively bound to their residential neighborhood—the youth, the nonworking housewife, the aged—all sorts of major social groups who are primarily locatable in the neighborhood and residence rather than in a job. I think this is one consideration we should bear in mind.

(*F. I.—methodology:* If the job is the start, you fan out to brothers, family, friends—a job-culture network which includes a variety of occupations, yet is a social and cultural unit.)

Hinkle: If you start with the job, say the Irish policeman, you'll find that the Irish policeman's brothers, family, friends, and associates would also be working. He's bound to have a brother in the transit, another that's a priest, another who works for Con Edison, and a fourth perhaps who works for the telephone company. Also he's going to have a sister who's married to somebody in the sheriff's office. So you get a network of possibilities. You get a job-culture group in which job refers to a variety of occupations, and yet they are social and cultural groups.

(*F. I.—work situation:* The job may not be as major in the worker's life as investigators of industry believe.)

Hinkle: I'm sorry I missed the last meeting. I'm not clear as to what extent my own experiences have been covered, but I would like to comment on my feelings about the role of the job in the total social and interpersonal environment of the individual. I'm approaching it from the point of view of an investigator from the outside, who comes with a view of the job situation as only being one aspect of this person's total life situation. One other thing, I think I detect a bias in most of those who write about the working man. They start with the work unit, with those people who are in the unit taken together, and with those who have to do with the management of this unit, and then they focus intensely upon how a change in working condition, administrative functions, or various manipulations that are carried on in the job seem to be relevant to the manifestation of behavior and health in the individual in it. One gets the impression in this way that this is really a major factor in their lives, whereas if you come at it from the point of view of those who work on the job, you see that the manipulations possible by management in organizational conditions don't look nearly as large to them as one might think.

(F. I.—work situation: Certain social groups concentrate in types of occupation situations which become part of a total way of life, and possibly not as important as other parts for their mental state.)

The thing that has struck us in working in New York City is: first of all, to a certain extent the people in the job select each other. Certain social groups, ethnic groups, as well as friendship groups, or family relative groups, tend to fall into the job situations, and, in effect, the job with all its measures becomes a part of their lives in which the manipulations of the managers, and the labor-management relationships, and changes and processes, don't look so important as they might seem. You have a good boss or bad boss, or a good group of working people, or changing conditions as a part of the way of business. What goes on in a job can be a source of expostulation among those who work there, a source of expression of feeling, sometimes a demonstration, but as one studies these people, you see that what goes on within their home and friendship groups often seems to be more related to the fluctuations in their mental state than what they're doing.

To me the job, the occupational situation, has been chiefly helpful in that when you make use of this feature within a complex social organization, such as New York City, the employment itself is not so much, the physical features of the employment are not so important, as that the job is a key to the type of people who work there. If one selects people who work in the transit system, Consolidated Edison, the telephone company, for example, one is selecting an Irish-American, German-American, Catholic working group. If one goes to the garment industry, one gets a different group; if one selects barbers, if one selects hospital orderlies, sanitation department workers, you get still other odd segments of the society, so that occupation would seem to me to be a social indicator. It's a segment of a life of the individuals who work there which in itself cannot be an entire indication as to what's going on with them, or necessarily the most important one.

(F. I.—work situation: Self-selection and time of entry into an occupation must be taken into account when investigating a work place.)

Illsley: I think this is a very important point in looking at a lot of work groups, that people are self-selected into them, and it depends to some extent when you begin to study them. I was thinking particularly as you were speaking of the salt fishing industry that we studied in Aberdeen. This isn't one of those fishing communities where father follows son; it's a very depressed industry in many ways, and I'd say the first feature of it is that people go into this, in general, who have found difficulty in obtaining and retaining employment in other jobs. This would be a feature, therefore, of the kind of people that you meet in the industry.

(F. I.—work situation: This type of occupation can influence the pattern of marital roles. Extended periods at sea by Aberdeen fishermen required complete role separation, while considerable overlap was characteristic of railway workers on shifts.)

Secondly, they go into it when they're fairly young, when they're single people, and I watched them dropping out of it. It's the kind of job where you're away for about three weeks on board ship; you come back and you have sixty hours at home between trips. This means that the family life of individuals in the industry is very restricted indeed, and the social life of this whole group depends greatly on the women in the group. But as they get married, and particularly as they have children, you begin to see individuals dropping out of the patrol fishing industry and going into another.

Now, these aren't just any individuals. These are quite clearly, from the personal histories that we have of them, people who, either from their own inclinations or from the pressure of their wives, are not prepared to carry on in this kind of industry when their situation changes. So if you study married men and older men in the salt fishing industry, you're studying a group who have been heavily selected along at least two dimensions, and who, to some extent aren't prepared to accept this kind of life. A research program will have to take this system of self-selection into account. I can think of another one where perhaps the process goes the other way—this is in our railway industry, which gives the working-class man very much more security than most industries do; it gives him super-annuation policies; that kind of thing. They go into it when they're young, and one of the things that we've noticed of these people is that they have a great deal of shift work, and the shift work again imposes a certain pattern on their family and marital activities. We categorized a whole series of occupations and individuals in terms of the degree of segregation of marital roles and found that in this particular industry there was an enormous amount of overlap between roles. It was the one working class occupation we felt which approached the kind of notion of a partnership marriage where people were doing things very much together, husband and wife, and had made joint decisions on all kinds of different things. Here, I think possibly the type of work that they're in has determined their marital relationship, whereas in the other instance, it might be the other way around. I think, therefore, one has to look very carefully, not only at the type of job, but into selection and the time they go into it.

Murphy: In this group, after your people are selected out, from social changes and from the disadvantages of the type of occupation, do they become stable workers in another occupation? You said they came in with histories of erratic employment, and do they maintain that? Do they work a little while in numerous categories?

(*F. I.—work situation:* Workers leaving the salted fish industry because of social demands are likely to hold stable jobs, while those remaining continue an erratic pattern, remaining in fishing, but changing connections.)

Illsley: No, I think the people that moved out of the fishing industry at this point would be the ones who were most likely to be able to hold down stable jobs, whereas the others remained in the industry.
Murphy: Then, do they leave and then come back?
Illsley: No, they don't. Once this kind of individual gets into the fishing industry, he doesn't move so much. Once you have the process of selection out, the more stable individuals, the others remain in. Their instability then takes a different form. It takes the form of moving around from one company to another, one firm to another, one beat to another, being late for the ship, and arriving when it's already departed, and so on, but they remain in the fishing industry because they can't hold down another job.

(*F. I.—work situation:* Job variability, rather than stability, may be preferred by some workers.)

Murphy: This suggests a variable that we didn't consider at all last week, and this is that job variability may have some satisfaction for certain types of people, that the newness, the lack of getting roots, can be one way that keeps them plugging along.

(F. I.—work situation: Two major categories in job selection demonstrated here: One where work is one aspect of cultural whole; the other which attracts similar personality types from different cultures. It suggests possibility that some types of work may attract workers having psychiatric disorders.)

A. Leighton: Dr. Hinkle has emphasized that work is one aspect of a cultural globule, and Dr. Illsley has emphasized the more atomic aspect, that certain jobs attract personality types who may come from rather different cultures, a kind of residual collection. It seems to me this is an important distinction that would suggest looking at the possibility of categorizing jobs, looking at them to see, in the first place, which of these two major categories they belong to, because the dynamics, the meaning of the job, and all the rest of it would be quite different probably, in these two types of situations. It also suggests the possibility that some types of work may attract people that we would categorize as having psychiatric disorders. I am thinking particularly of the picture of the fishing industry, which sounded as if it attracted psychopathic personalities. Is this so or not?

Illsley: It is so, yes.

A. Leighton: There may be other jobs that attract people with one or another liability from a mental health point of view, but the job provides a kind of niche.

(F. I.—work situation: Both social and job characteristic selection factors operate for most jobs, making hazardous the use of a work situation when generalization or representation is desired.)

Hinkle: I think both points are true in almost every job. If we turn to the telephone operator, for example, in New York City, at the present time, one can be quite sure that this occupation will attract girls who have no more than a high school education, and often somewhat less, and who are either Protestant or Catholic, but not Jewish; second generation Irish or Italian in general, with some Czechs and Slavs, and Negroes (in the telephone offices the Negroes are in numbers proportional to their numbers in the community). Within this group are women and girls who have some work because they are of communities, and of groups, in which their families and friends have worked for this industry.

You will find that out of 100 who begin to work at the age of 17 or 18, not more than ten remain at the age of 27 or 28. These ten are a highly selected group who do not or are not able to follow the preferred pattern in their social group, which is to marry the man who can provide the chief income while the wife stays home to be a mother of a family. They are either single women or women who, for one reason or another, decide to be career women, and the selection from this group is quite the opposite from what one finds for the career man. Of the men who come, 80 percent of them will stay for a career.

But to think of these characteristics of jobs—it's the experience in large corporations that the sales group is always rather different from the other groups because these men prefer to work on commission, prefer the change and challenge of this, and more or less reject or have difficulty in accepting such things as pension plans and tenure. At other levels you find groups such as the longshoremen in New York City, or the people in Actors' Equity; in both of these groups anywhere from 30 to 80-90 percent of the people at any one time are unemployed, and yet, for various, chiefly personal reasons, this particular type of employment is so much preferred to any other type of activity that they will not get out of it.

The possibility of using an industrial group, both as an indicator of a social group and as a selector of people by means of social processes, is a very attractive one that can readily be made use of. It has the opposite effect in that it's very hazardous to make any assumption about generalization or representation to any sort of employment.

(*F. I.—work situation:* Isn't the intention to use the work place as one of many systems in which the individual operates, and not as the central place for the research?)

Freydberg: I don't think the purpose of going into the work situation was in terms of a particular work situation as the focus for moving out, rather we were thinking in terms of various systems that the individual moves into in his environment, of which one is the work situation, the family another, etc. The thought was not to concentrate the research in a work organization as the center. Am I correct about that?

D. Leighton: We're trying to think of meaningful groupings of people, isn't that what it is? Wherever it is?

Freydberg: Or meaningful to the individual?

D. Leighton: That's right.

(*F. I.—work situation:* Previous emphasis was on work environment. Now we are adding the selective factor, and when the work situation is part of a cultural work component.)

A. Leighton: But in our previous discussion of the work situation our emphasis has been on the effect of the environment on the individual, whereas this one is bringing into play the selective factor; also what goes on in the work situation is only a part of what the job means to the people having this membership in a cultural work group component. These are both things which I think we didn't touch on before.

(*F. I.—work situation:* An occupation study of women showed that after five years 50% had changed to jobs not requiring similar skills. The criterion was flexibility to allow for family affairs, demonstrating the over-riding strength of this rather than work conditions.)

Illsley: This became very clear to me in looking at the occupations of

women over a five-year period. I took their premarital occupations or
their early married occupations before they had children and looked at
them about five years later and found a tremendous changeover in
occupations. Of the women of the later period, well over half of them
weren't working in the same occupation, nor at an occupation that
required the same types of skills as they had on the previous occasion.
You'd find them in this occupation not for work reasons alone; they
moved into it mainly in order to give themselves flexibility for the
handling of their family affairs. The fact that you find them in this
particular occupation is an indication of the strength of their family ties
and the strength of their family commitments. In studying them one
would have to take this very much into account, rather than the work
situation itself and the conditions of job. This was what meant a great
deal to them, the family, rather than the work situation. I think this
bears on your other point of how different the meaning of work is to
different social groups.

(*F. I.—work situation:* All members of an ethnic group in a work
situation do not necessarily belong to the same social system away from
work. Investigation is possible to determine the overlap patterns.)

Murphy: I wonder if any of these selective factors that we've
mentioned, such as ethnic group, have variance to another social system
of interaction. If a certain number of these people in the telephone
company are all of common ethnic background, we can say that we
know certain things about them because they belong to an ethnic
group. But we're using group, I think, in a very different sense from
that which would mean a social system, where all of the Negroes in the
telephone office, for example, would, outside the telephone office, also
form a social system because they are Negro and do not live in the same
neighborhood as whites, and so on. It may be that that happens in
certain instances, but in our first meeting you were making the point

that there was surprising diversity among the people even though they were Negro—some were Jamaican Negroes, etc. It would be an investigatable point, I think, and it might lead us into some understanding of how the personnel in one social group overlap with the personnel in another, but I don't think we could presume it.

(F. I.—work situation: Is a saliency factor determinable among work and other social systems that would permit an ordering?)

(F. I.—work situation: Even within an ethnic group in a work situation, there can be considerable diversity of social systems outside, but it is not utterly random.)

Hinkle: Well, there is a surprising diversity but this is not utterly random. I think that the point here is that the occupational group is one facet of a group of interrelated social systems. If you go to a group of men who are, let us say, working in the advertising industry, you find that these people, in spite of a considerable diversity from person to person, nonetheless are inclined to have roughly the same sort of education, work in sort of a limited number of associations in an area in New York, live in definable areas around New York City, and are married to women of rather definable social groups, so that this is a key to getting into a great many interlocking things. This group, I think, would not at all overlap with my group of telephone operators, or only very little. It is true also that there are variations among the Negro groups and within a Negro group. In a community of Negro women, you would see in their household relationships and in their interpersonal relationships a considerable variation on a family-to-family basis within the range that's possible for people of this social community, and in this particular group within our society, so that there are both variations, but not infinite variation.

Freydberg: Is there any saliency factor among the different systems that the work situation can be contrasted with, the family situation, for instance? Any way of ordering these on the basis of some sort of hierarchy of influence or importance?

(Among telephone operators studied, certain family events would be more crucial to health than changes affecting work.)

Hinkle: Yes, I would say that a change in supervisor, or in income, or in some aspect of the job, such as the shift-over, which has been recently going on to direct-distance dialing and which has put a lot of girls who had formerly been long distance operators into information operating which they find less interesting, are even less pertinent to health than what happens to the husband or a sister, or a mother, or a failure of conjunction between two sets of values, such as I mentioned in the terms of the Jamaican Negro man married to an American Negro woman. I think you could approach this methodologically by getting a group of people and setting up, *a priori*, certain categories and things that you were going to measure or count, and I think you would probably find that, in general for this group, minor variations in the job are less crucial in terms of behavior or bodily function than threats to home or disturbances arising within the family.

(*F. I.—work situation:* Saliency of the work situation is greater for men than women, and probably varies for men according to social class.)

Langner: You've been talking about women. I think everybody would accept the fact that men's work role is more crucial to their ego image than women's where they must achieve a balance between family and work roles. Depending on social class, too, I think, the work role looms larger or smaller in the man's life, so again, every time you take a step, you have to say: well, hold on, let's look at the sexes, let's look at the class.

Hinkle: It would have to be an open question for each new group. I was merely making the point that I think these things could be ordered in degree of importance, and this order could be tested, its relationship to manifestations of disturbance, a particular mood, or psychoses.

(*F. I.—work situation:* Place of interview may affect saliency of system. The same individuals appear to stress what is related to that location.)

Whyte: One thing we might consider is where the interviewing is conducted. Dubin a while back published a study that suggested that those of us who'd been studying relations of people within the plant were overemphasizing the importance of the work situation. In his studies, people seemed little concerned with this, and much more concerned with home and community. But the study was carried out through interviews in the home and in the community, and I can't prove this, but I have the impression from the reports of field workers that if you interviewed the same individuals in the plant, they seem very concerned about everything that's going on in the plant, and everything outside seems quite remote. If you interviewed them in the home, the same people, why they'd be much concerned about the home, the plant is very remote and not of much concern. We would have to be careful if we were moving in on this question to take this possible separation of spheres in people's minds and feelings into account.

(*F. I.—work situation:* Attraction for particular groups can cause a differential selection. Being repelled also can, as the telephone company's reputation of not hiring Jewish operators.)

Chein: I think there are a variety of dynamic factors involved here: (1) With regard to the differential selection that takes place; in part, I think one can attribute this to the fact that certain kinds of people are attracted, but I think it's also true that other kinds of people are apt to be repelled. The absence of Jews as telephone operators, I think, is, in part, a matter of history. When Jewish girls would have been very much attracted to it, they were not attracted because of, at least a belief, that the telephone company wouldn't take them because they were Jewish, and so, in terms of the public image, they were being repelled rather than not wanting to go into this work.

(F. I.—work situation: A vital determinant in the individual's selection and satisfaction of occupation are his degrees of freedom in making a choice and in molding the job itself to his needs. The extent to which the job is integrated or segregated from the rest of his life is probably related to this; the less freedom of choice and action the greater the segregation.)

A good deal, I think, is also involved in the issue of the general economic situation, and the relative degrees of freedom that an individual has in choice of moving, which leads him to one job rather than another job. If he hasn't got the freedom to move, then his personal predilections won't make too much difference. I don't think that it's ever a situation of a total lack of freedom, but, in effect, it becomes an issue of how much the individual has to impose on his environment by way of forcing it to meet his needs. I think this is also true within the job situation, in terms of the degree to which he can mold it to his needs, mold it by having selected people that he can associate with more intimately, mold it by in some way transforming the job from one set of specifications to his own specifications, not necessarily verbally articulating this, but nevertheless, he does with the job what he wants to do rather than what anybody else expects him to do. The degree of freedom in doing this would make a heck of a difference in terms of what kind of a picture he will find within job settings. I also note, just to shift for a moment, that it seems pretty clear to me that one can find a complete continuum between the job as an essentially segregated portion of one's life, and a job as something that is completely integrated in one's life from the point of view of there being virtually no connection between what happens in the job and what happens as soon as one leaves the plant or the place of work. Conversely, wherever one happens to be, one is constantly working at one's job. Whether at home or at a social gathering, the company that's there are there because this is in some way related to one's job and to whom one talks to, to how one talks, what one talks about, what one thinks about, what one talks about to one's wife and to all the rest of them.

Now, I suspect that this kind of integration of the job into one's total life pattern, or its essential segregation from the rest of one's life pattern is not unrelated to the degrees of freedom which one experiences in selecting the job or in molding it to one's desires.

In effect, the more one is in a situation where one has no choice, I expect that this would be a condition conducive to segregating the job experience. The more freedom of choice and freedom of action one has, the more the job would be integrated into the rest of one's life because one's job is, in effect, and expression of one's way of doing things and so on.

(*F. I.—family:* Role segmentation in lower blue-collar families is such that husbands do not talk to wives or help with children. Variation in segmentation is as great in the family system as in jobs.)

Langner: This is something that cuts across lots of our functions then. To mention a few, Komarovsky's study of environment shows that in working-class families the role is segmented, husbands don't talk to wives. Husbands talk to people they meet in a bar, who may not necessarily be close friends, and this isn't the unstable factory worker necessarily, it's lower blue collar, and the wives talk to their mothers. There's virtually no relationship between husbands and wives as we might know it in the middle-class family. They don't discuss the children, that's the wife's problem, and the wife does not discuss the husband's job. It seems to me that role segmentation varies strongly not only on the job, but with the male and female role also. We see the husband doing a little bit of dish-washing and not worrying about loss of status in the middle-class family.

(*F. I.—family:* A further complication is found in the Midtown data which show a diminishing same-sex identification in more recent generations.)

The only clue we had in our Midtown questionnaire was, as we went up in generation, to a certain extent more girls said they took after father and more boys said they took after mother. The boys who took after mother had a higher impairment risk, whereas the girls who took after father had a lowered impairment risk. I don't know what it means, but I don't think there's any doubt about this finding as we took four generations. The sex differentials, the self-image of the person, and the trend to similar sex identification, as much as this questionnaire tapped it, was definitely diminishing. It seems to me this definitely makes for a problem if you're going to sample occupations because their meanings are going to relate to the social level, to the skills involved, and with the whole style of role learning, which may be segmented or non-segmented. *Chein:* Well, I think that's one reason why we're in a rather helpless position, and I'm not sure that we can do more than be helpless about it. But if we can detect what the dynamics of this are, then it seems to me we're not completely helpless because our attention then gets directed, not to what's essentially insignificant, but to what establishes the situation.

(*F. I.—family:* A heavily structured sex-role differentiation allows little freedom and requires greater personal forces to act in opposition.)

The same within-the-sex role differentiation, insofar as this is very heavily structured by the culture, allows an individual relatively few degrees of freedom about it, and one can then look upon this fact as an impingement of an environment on him, something that he's helpless about. For him to be able to overcome this requires a great deal more force, and this works both ways, both in terms of where one would expect idiosyncratic personality motivation or where factors can enter in more strongly than in situations where there are more degrees of freedom for this to happen. Or, conversely, if an individual is acting contrary to norms, one could deduce that the idiosyncratic personality motivation factors must be much more potent than where the individual is yielding to the social force, where it's a matter of environment rather than of person.

(Less pathology is indicated for a Negro boy in Harlem involved in narcotics than a white boy in Riverdale. The former is moving with a social force, the latter against it.)

Well, again let me take an example from the Glover (phonetic) Dictionary. I think I've got a substantial amount of evidence to indicate that for Negro boys in Harlem to become involved with narcotics is much less indicative of personal psychopathology than for a white boy in Riverdale. In effect, the Negro boy in Harlem is moving with a social force; the white boy in Riverdale is moving against the social force, and so I think what we've got to do is learn to look at these things both in terms of forces acting on the person, and in terms of opportunities for the person to act within the set of social forces.

(F. I.—environment: The "fit" in terms of background, experience, and temperament of an individual and his situation in life seems related to manifestations of illness. Generalizations based on characteristics of many facets of society are difficult.)

Hinkle: In our own studies, one of the things that has guided us toward taking circumscribed environments and studying them intensively has been our feeling that, in general terms, one of the most important determinants of health seems to be the fit between the particular person and the ecological niche that he happens to occupy. If a person is by background and experience, by temperament, and so far as this is available, by his personal choice, well-suited to the particular situation in life in which he finds himself, and not motivated nor driven to attempt to move out of this, it has been our general impression that such people are content doing the job that they do and show relatively fewer manifestations of illness than those who do not fit very closely or who fit very poorly with that particular niche. Yet, at the same time, we've had the feeling that some of those who were doing poorly and who fitted very poorly into the particular niche that they occupied might have been healthy had they been in other situations more suited to their particular needs. So I do believe that what both of you have said about the very special characteristics of the socially determined features of the many little facets in our society that people can occupy, are not important, in the sense that you can't necessarily generalize on these things, that the fit between persons and situations has to be studied both in terms of the sophisticated knowledge of the meaning of this type of situation and a sophisticated understanding of the particular needs of the individual.

(F. I.—work situation: We need to look as well at aspects of the job situation that may or may not be compatible with the individual's personality needs.)

Whyte: It seems to me in looking at this trend, we have to look not only at the social role played by the individual in the community, the family, social class, so on, nor, on the other hand, simply at the industry where he's working, especially in our telephone industry, but at certain aspects of the job situation that may or may not be compatible with the individual's personality.

I was recently talking to Harrison Trice at Cornell about some preliminary work he'd done with night watchmen on the Cornell campus. Cornell is a big organization with lots of types of jobs; this is quite a unique job in its interaction or rather lack of it. He found that these individuals tended to be of a paranoid type; they tend to be suspicious of people and don't care to have them around very much. This seemed a pretty good job for this type of individual to have.

It may have something in common with a study I saw years ago of the oil industry, a particular job of engine operator. This required the man to remain practically all his working day in a shed where six large engines kept hammering away. They created a tremendous noise, but also there was nobody else there. When I came down to try to interview him about the noise, we found that the men who were there and wanted to stay there had grown up on farms, and it was a sort of a family farm where you could be off on your own for a large part of the day. The boys who had grown up in town and were used to some kind of gang associations might have to go through this job because it was one of the lower jobs, but they struggled to get out of it; they were very unhappy.

I think, even among jobs that appear on the surface to be the same job, you have to make discriminations in personality requirements, e.g., selling in a department store. I recall from Eliot Chapple's study where he contrasts the job of the girl at the notions counter with the girl in the millinery department; he reports that these girls might be equally good sales persons, but they just were not interchangeable. The girl at the notions counter would have interactions with a large number of people during the day, but of very brief duration, whereas the girl in the millinery department would interact with a few individuals and would have to maintain interaction over a long period of time while the lady figured out did she or did she not want to buy this hat.

(*F. I.—work situation:* Certain personalities may prefer a specific type of job. However, the job experience itself may be the cause of preference.)

Now, this is just anecdotal, but he described a situation where things were slack in the notions department, and the management consulted Chapple about transferring this crack sales girl in notions to millinery, and he advised against it, predicting that she would not do a good selling job and that she would be unhappy. They transferred her anyway and the result was that she did not do a good selling job and she was unhappy. Now, this is not evidence of course, it's just a dramatic example, but I think it suggests something that we need to consider in looking at a work situation. You can make discriminations among different types of jobs, not only in terms of the attraction they may have for people of certain class backgrounds, and men versus women, and so on, but in terms of the interactional requirements of the jobs.

Freydberg: This goes back to an earlier point made by Dr. Illsley about the job also being a certain influence on other systems. I think Kurt Lewin in a way sort of epitomized it when he was talking about the eating habits of people. He felt to a large extent that they didn't eat what they'd like, but they liked what they ate.

I think a job can form a person's preference. I think there are other instances where selective factors work.

Whyte: This would be interesting to study, that it works both ways. Presumably the job has a selective pull or repulsion according to the personality characteristics of individuals, but once you get in the job, if you make any sort of adjustment to the job, this must, I assume, change what you like.

(*F. I.—work situation:* Research on a group of nuns discloses a tendency for this selection by one daughter of a recently arrived

Catholic family. Other daughters' occupations were principally semi-skilled or unskilled clerical or factory jobs. It suggests a means of determining the available choices and basis for decision.)

Hinkle: I think this also is an investigatable question. It would seem to me that for any social group the society does provide certain possibilities, and that these can, in a way, be defined. For example, we've recently been studying a group of nuns who are in a diocesan teacher's college, and we were very interested in trying to find out what young women at the present time would go into this sort of thing. We have, of course, found that the vast majority of them come from strongly Roman Catholic families, but interestingly enough, nearly all are from Roman Catholic families very recently arrived in this country, in which the value of becoming a nun, of sending a girl to the Church, is still high in the minds of both parents and their children. This is much less true among equally strongly Catholic families who had been here for several generations.

But quite aside from this, only one daughter from a family of several daughters would choose this. As you discussed with these girls the occupational choices of their sisters, you could see that these are not infinite, that their sisters become skilled or semiskilled factory workers, or they may become clerical workers of the lowest level. They may occasionally become sales people; there have been a few of them who have become domestics, service workers, but there are not an infinite number of possibilities for these girls. Within this range both social and psychological factors compelled them to this choice rather than one of the others open to them. Now, I'm sure the same phenomenon that could provide an opening for this sort of maneuver could provide an opening for making an estimate of the number of choices available to people in a certain situation and an evaluation of why they happened to choose this.

(F. I.—environment: Jahoda proposed studying an environment by identifying those fitting in it best. In this way you can learn about the setting.)

Chein: In this general connection, I'd like to mention an idea that Marie Jahoda had about an approach to a study of social environments which would proceed by first identifying individuals who fit best into a given social content. By studying the properties of these individuals, one can take it as axiomatic that the environment is one that is best accommodated to the individuals who fit it best. Her notions ranged all the way from relatively small social contexts, things such as a job or college, to the national character as one would be able to define it in terms of a given national setting. What kinds of individuals are most comfortable in a nation? If one knows their problems, then one knows something about the properties of the setting.

Langner: If you look at it through time, this is to be a longitudinal study, and you want to talk about fitting into an environment, I don't know if five years would be long enough to see this kind of change. I'm sure there will be several short-term changes. I will give just one example from my work interviewing parents. It's very obvious that the work role is connected with the parental role, but if you ask parents whether the things they do have any connection with child-rearing practices, they'll throw up their hands and say: "Are you crazy? I don't mix my work and my family; you know, I'm not training my kid to do what I do, I want him to be better than I am."

Aberle has a very good article on this in which he talks about the unconscious training of the children for certain types of behavior. It would be very foolish for a father to train his son to have a lot of initiative if the father's occupation is to push a wheelbarrow of cement and to go along a 2 x 12 plank with it. If he had a lot of initiative he might just run right off it. It just doesn't fit. Still, let's say he's given some ideas about keeping on the plank to the child, but when it comes time for that boy at 17 to work, he is faced with automation and various other things; there's not as much of his father's kind of job left. The father's mental health may be affected because he has sort of fitted him in an unfit way, so that, through time, this being fit in a particular environment may rebound, even on individuals, particularly from generation to generation.

These mothers and fathers may be emotionally upset because they make a connection between their failure to train their children in a certain way. This may occur even during a five-year period; you will find that men and women who are moving into new jobs are becoming upset by the fact that their own values are out of line with the job situation. When we think over-all that those who fit best in the environment are going to be the best adjusted, and if the environment is a changing phenomenon, it seems to me you've got to have a new set of definitions that refer to flexibility.

(F. I.—environment: If rigid, people were happiest, this tells a major property of the situation. A judgment of trouble if change occurs is a deduction of the effect of a certain direction of change.)

Chein: The proposition though wasn't that they'd be best adjusted. The proposition was: From studying the properties of individuals who fit best, one can explore the characteristics of the situation. In your example, if it turns out that highly rigid, inflexible people are the happiest and most content and least desirous of a change, and so on in their situation, this tells you that a major property of the situation is something that doesn't call for adjustment, patience, initiative, etc. You might then well deduce that if the situation were to change, these would be the individuals who would be in the most trouble, but you would also be deducing a direction of change in environment that would produce the trouble.

(F. I.—environment: The stability of the situation has an effect. Among

a group of uprooted Chinese left in circumstances of uncertainty, the least symptomatic were shallow in attachments, able to live fluidly, and almost sociopathic. For most people, however, the environment in middle years does not change drastically.)

Hinkle: Considerations of this sort led us a few years ago to study a group of Chinese. We had first studied groups of people who lived in rather fixed and unchanging social situations in the United States for many years of middle life, and we found these people to be the least symptomatic, the least ill of these people in stereotype routines who lacked security. We then turned to this group of Chinese who had not only a vast amount of both social and cultural change within their own society, but had been uprooted and left over here for ten years in a situation of uncertainty. Using the same indicators of health, we found that many of the Chinese who had been least symptomatic displayed a shallowness of personal attachment, a shallowness of attachment to goals, and an ability to live in fluid situations such that, under other circumstances, one might have said that they were almost sociopathic individuals.

I think that what Dr. Chein was saying is that fish do well in water. It does seem to be that the people who have few symptoms are, in general, going to fit rather well in the particular situation in which they find themselves all the time. It is true that you can find people in whom the life situation changes to a major degree, but, by and large, over a period of middle life, for a large number of these people, the broad social features of the environment are not going to change much.

(*F. I.—environment:* The skills of Puerto Rican women coming to New York fit into the garment industry, but an equivalent to it did not occur for the men. This caused difficulty for the more crucial family environment.)

Murphy: I wonder if some of the things that we're saying about fit aren't very well illustrated by Oscar Handlin's view of Puerto Rican women coming into New York City, where many of them have gone into garment factories. Now, here's a national group that went into a particular occupation, but I don't think we could say in this instance that a national character dimension is involved. I don't think we can say it's a personality feature, it's not Chapple's notions or the millinery type, but it's probably that they have the prerequisite skills based on the kind of training that they've had before coming to New York City, and there was a good place in the environment for them to fit immediately and become economically valuable. But this, then, caused considerable difficulty in their families because Puerto Rican men didn't have a comparable fit. So you would expect, over time, especially since we're looking at a group of women, for this to have a kind of backlash, and that you would soon find them in a situation jarring to the rest of their environment, their crucial environment at any rate.

(F. I.—work situation: The ambitions of the worker and judgment of his qualifications by others is related to fit and psychopathology.)

Michael: As we go around the table and talk about fit, I'm thinking about patients that I've seen, people that really have trouble with their jobs. One particular one was referred to me because he couldn't hold a job. His father was a successful industrialist, a director-vice president of a division of a large company. The patient's ambition was to be just that. Whenever he went to try for jobs, it was usually with a large company like Minnesota Mining. He usually applied for a job that called for recent college graduates, though he was ten years out of college and didn't quite graduate. He passed the screening tests and went for an interview, and they always decided that he was fit for a salesman, though his ambition was to get into administration and become director of the factory, president, or something like this. The point that I'm making is that an important factor of this fit is the ambition of the worker, and how well he is able to fulfill it in relation to what society, the factory, or his employer think he is suited for. This might be a fruitful area to look into defining psychopathology.

(*F. I.—situation:* A worker's expectations can be viewed as contributing to goodness to fit.)

Freydberg: You could subsume expectation under this idea of fit, I would say it would be part of that kind of general category.

I wonder if I could jump here into another one that I want to point at Dr. Hinkle, the question of degrees of freedom. Did you find any data at all that would indicate that jobs with less degrees of freedom were more constricting in this sense, or were any more inclined to affect mental health, than those that had more degrees of freedom?

(*F. I.—environment:* In this country, when people believe their freedom of choice is restricted, they are ill more often. Actually for any social class, freedom of choice is far less than it may seem.)

Hinkle: Well, I haven't had as much experience with this as some of the anthropologists. I think that they were the ones who first pointed out to me that the feeling of a need for freedom of choice is a feature of some societies, of Western societies in general, and of American societies in particular.

In conclusion, we are confronted with several compelling research questions: How do we best study job-cultures? How do we go beyond social class to more dynamic formulations of social processes and mental health? How do we account for jobs as need-meeting niches? In a preventive sense, how are people best fitted to a niche that would maximize health and minimize illness?

Some Special Methodological
Problems in Studying Urban Areas

BERTON H. KAPLAN, Ph.D.

Contributors

John Gulick, Ph.D.	Herbert Gans, Ph.D.
Alexander H. Leighton, M.D.	Nicholas Freydberg, Ph.D.
Jane Murphy, Ph.D.	Paul V. Gump, Ph.D.

The focus in Seminar 10 was on conceptual and methodological problems related to research on social process in an urban area. The results of this session are summarized [1] in the following statement:

THE COMMUNITY APPROACH IN AN URBAN SETTING

The identification of an environment on a continuum of integration-disintegration, and the measurement of the influence of this variable on the mental health of residents, has previously been done in rural areas where one finds more or less self-contained, geographic communities of moderate size in which the bulk of individuals work and are acquainted with one another. The present plan is to select units, probably facing

[1] This summary was written by Nicholas Freydberg, Ph.D.

blocks, within and representative of certain census tracts that will be chosen on the basis of criteria available from public records such as the U.S. Census. On the basis of this data it probably will be possible to parallel roughly the criteria employed for classification of rural communities in Nova Scotia as integrated, disintegrated, and intermediate. The question is whether these urban units are communities in the same way and as essential in the lives of their inhabitants.

Skepticism was voiced about the cognizance of community generally. In a social sense, Levittown, a suburb of Philadelphia (recently studied by one participant, Herbert Gans), was seen as a community by most of its residents only insofar as they had a few friends in the area and participated peripherally in one or two organizations. Politically, unity was limited to occasional protests if taxes rose, and beyond that it would be hard to trace any community impact. Another participant (John Gulick,) who had done research in Tripoli, in another culture, did not find any over-all sense of community as occurs in Nova Scotia; in Tripoli people cohered only when threatened by outsiders. This has been seen in New York City in the unified neighborhood protests to relocation because of the requirements of the urban renewal program, when people appear to feel that they live in areas that mean a great deal to them.

The relevant dimension in a community may be the extent to which its residents are interdependent. In this regard, some diminution of this may be occurring even in rural communities where many of the responsibilities formerly borne by the village are now relegated to larger political units and to highly professionalized talent, as is seen in road building and protection. In Nova Scotia, a community was not identified by "we-ness" but as a collection of people living together geographically, interdependent economically and for effective law and order, for education, and for protection against disease, fire, and acts of God. All this can be accomplished without anyone necessarily feeling devoted to the community. Functionally these things get done in integrated communities, but misfire in disintegrated ones.

Will this kind of interdependence exist in New York City in the blocks selected as the areas for investigation, where health, transit, educational, and protection services emanate from outside, and most likely the wage earner's work situation is located somewhere else? The absence of garbage scattered outside apartment houses on Park Avenue, in contrast to nearby areas in Harlem, was suggested as evidence of interdependence and functioning in the city. Sharply diverging here was the view that even the worst neighborhoods in New York City could not be labeled as disintegrated for at least 90 percent of the people living in them were law-abiding but simply were unable to defend themselves as well as Park Avenue residents.

If the research decision is to focus on where urban residents live in order to determine its influence on them, then there may be no need to define it as a community. The concern is with the kind of interaction that occurs outside of the household; this defines the kind of environment or "community." The lack of interaction in the case of the thirty or so neighbors on a Queens street who did nothing to aid a woman being murdered, not even calling the police, indicates the level of functional interdependence to expect on that block.

On the other hand, if the research is not committed to a fixed community, the environment of the urban individual offers an alternative. In the city, unlike the self-contained community, the place of work is rarely near one's residence, and this often is true of the location of kin and friends. Function and interdependence are certainly diluted compared to the rural village, and in fact might not be with one's neighbors, but with others outside. We need to know a good deal more about how environmental forces impinge on this person. In Tripoli an adaptation of Kevin Lynch's technique was employed to locate the meaningful environment for a respondent. He was asked to make a map of where he usually went in the city and what it meant to him. Possibly it could be determined in the survey questionnaire by asking where his friends live, etc.

If there is a research commitment, it is to a social process unit that qualifies as a social system meaningful to the individual and to which the concept of integration-disintegration can apply. What remains to be determined is whether the residential neighborhoods play a sufficiently significant role in urbanite life for most people. If not, it may be necessary to follow the individual outward.

BEHAVIOR SETTINGS AS INDICATORS OF INTERACTION

The Barker behavior settings measures showed in Nova Scotia a high correlation between a large number of these settings and well-integrated communities, and between few settings and disintegrated communities. It raises the possibility of obtaining numerical scores by independent means for determining the degree to which this phenomena is present. Recent research by Barker and Gump, titled *Big School, Little School* and employing this technique, suggests some parallels with urban-rural differences. In the small school all must participate, but the greater number of students in the large school allows fewer to do so, and many become observers rather than participants. When the density of the population rises, the chance of any one person taking a position at the center is reduced. A characteristic side effect in the large school is a group of "outsiders," amounting to as many as 35 percent, who don't do much of anything, and it may account for the increase in dropouts for the rate in the large school is higher. As for consequences for mental health, it may make for a considerable difference, for nonparticipation encourages detachment, which is associated with pathology, and the dropouts support this contention. It is tempting to conjecture whether this is comparable with the urban dweller's removal from participation in many of the needs and services that form the basis for interdependence and relatedness in small communities. An assumption to be aware of here is that participation is being associated with mental health. A study of students in Colorado schools at the upper end of a participation scale showed a dichotomy. Some according to psychological tests were very outgoing and others were isolates who used activity as a protective shell.

How can one employ the behavior setting technique in a city? In the small town, Barker took every setting where people interacted and could just about manage it. Individuals in the city could be asked about their itineraries: where they went and why, with the view of winnowing it down to their meaningful environment. The problem then becomes one of evolving a rationale for segregation of these settings. In Nova Scotia the settings studied were those in which the same people interacted in order to get at the relative amount of disruption.

The sheer number of behavior settings on a block might be a worthwhile way of describing the geographic units in the city that are studied, but it does not tell us what these mean to those going in and out of them. The number of acquaintances you have and the number of organizations you belong to are not a solid base, it's the quality of relationships that count. A combination of possibilities was suggested. The area could be studied, it has certain qualities, some of the residents interact in the settings and others do not. Along with this, a random sample of the respondents for the area are selected and their environments are investigated. Perhaps, too, from this data a line can be drawn for a 50 percent environment, that is, where 50 percent of the people spend 50 percent of their abroad time within these limits. It becomes a double task. When looking at the circumscribed area, the question you're answering is about the area (or the community) in which people interact, and not the individual. The second question deals with the effective community or environment or interactions of people, which may or may not be congruent with the area under investigation.

SUITABILITY OF INTEGRATION-DISINTEGRATION
CONCEPT TO CITY

The interest of CPSP is in the relationship of integrated and disintegrated social systems to mental health. The environment of the urban disintegrated unit is not known and its determination probably will require participant observation. Some doubt was expressed that a whole area could be labeled integrated or disintegrated; mental illness undoubtedly will be found but it may have little to do with the culture of the block if only because the housing shortage has forced a heterogeneity in the population. While to the casual observer an area or block may appear to be homogeneous, it may not be so to the residents. For example, one section in Harlem has the reputation of being occupied wholly by transient families displaced time and again by housing projects, but investigators found that 40 percent have lived there seven years or more.

It was suggested that the term disintegration may be inappropriate since it assumes that there was some degree of integration initially, whereas there may have been no other system to start with. Moreover, effects may be rather a consequence of nonintegration rather than disintegration. The definition of disintegration as employed by the Cornell program in social psychiatry is presumed to cover unintegrated or nonintegrated areas and is not intended to imply a previous state. The determining factor for designation might well be a lack of interdependence or feeling that this is so when there is a need for it. The notion may not be applicable to the city without some reinterpretation. It applies to geographic areas that have certain functions of survival and self-perpetuation to perform, and integration or disintegration refers to the effectiveness of this interdependence in carrying out these functions. A community that is performing its social or behavioral functions is effectively providing some resources and is able to change certain deleterious circumstances, and there is a correlation with mental health if communities are arranged along a continuum in this regard.

The effect may be due to the kind of interface each individual experiences, which in an integrated community is benign but which in a disintegrated one is noxious. This quality of interface (which is not necessarily a property of a block or of a social system) may be translatable to the study of the urban environment, and comparisons become available once more is learned about the types of interface that are benign and noxious. Possibly this can be distilled initially by choosing census tract areas in the city comparable in criteria with the integrated and disintegrated communities in Nova Scotia where interface is known and by basing this study on the quality of interface in these tracts rather than in terms of community integration or disintegration. Interface is still analogous to living in an integrated community, and in the plan proposed it will result in some people living in the tract who really operate in a number of different ones, but interface is not necessarily geographically circumscribed for it refers to the relations individuals have with their social environment wherever that may be.

THE FUNCTION OF PARTICIPANT OBSERVATION

In Nova Scotia, participant observers working with key informants were the principal means employed for determining the integration and disintegration of communities. At times during the discussion it was mentioned that it was likely that this method would be needed to deal with a number of questions regarding the applicability of the concept to urban areas that are selected on the basis of public record criteria comparable with data on Nova Scotia communities identified as integrated, disintegrated, or intermediate. One such question was whether these urban sectors were sufficiently homogeneous to permit such a generalization. The afternoon session directed attention at the specific activities that would be suitable for observation and useful for the research objectives.

The participant observer can spot the individuals who have been interviewed and see what goes on when they are on the street and elsewhere, providing by this means a traceable connection with the interview. He can locate the focal points of the area's activities. It may be of value to have someone observe things that otherwise would be missed, such as a failure to mention the storekeeper when queried about neighborhood interaction, and this type of thing lends itself also to validating the questionnaire responses. One group of suggestions dealt with the use of key informants; several might be found on each block who would be in an appropriate position to pick up things which would be difficult to do in the interview, and these people might even be substituted for the trained observers. Doubt, however, was expressed of the desirability of placing too great a dependence on this source as key informants usually have only a piece of reality, and it would be misleading to attempt to generalize from it. Caution was expressed about unplanned observation; a carefully prepared design is needed to direct a focus on activities that have a meaning for the objectives of the research, that is, that are related to mental health, and to insure comparability across areas. If participant observation is to be used, spotting the sample of 500 all over the city becomes inadvisable; it is necessary to concentrate in only a few areas and to go deeper into these.

Behavior settings may prove the basis for organizing planned observation, for more than just the location of the settings is likely to be needed. Settings have different uses; it may be necessary to identify these, and also the people who interact in them rather than obtain only a straight count. Measures of the quality of the interaction and its length may be advisable. Behavior settings themselves tend to determine the kind of behavior; an absence of interaction in an elevator is hardly unusual. Knowledge of the kind of behavior to expect can be useful for it provides a baseline for measuring whether the behavior of a particular individual is dysfunctional. Considering the number of settings potentially possible in an urban area, it may be necessary to subsample these, but it must be done with sufficient knowledge to stratify within the population of settings in order to insure an appropriate representation. In Nova Scotia there was a sorting of healthy from nonhealthy settings; the amount of time people spent in each was determined; and a picture of their social field was obtained in this way. Along with this, a status-role concept was formed for residents in terms of their activities in order to determine whether in interaction these were appropriately perceived. The idea was to be able to say whether, in general, segments of interaction in the community met expectations or didn't and thereby caused disruption.

PROBLEMS IN THE USE OF BEHAVIOR SETTINGS

The work required for behavior setting measurements, according to one discussant, is so enormous that it is not feasible in the city unless it can be telescoped by key informants providing the essential information about the community settings, the actors, and the behavior, which then would enable the mapping out of the community in a relatively brief time. Even so, to make observations relatively objective and reproducible, you need to concentrate a number of independent raters at a setting and to check on the extent to which they are in agreement. This procedure is needed also to guard against the danger of contamination of the independent and dependent variables, for these interpretations of setting are closely related to the mental health condition of the community. In short, the more objective, reproducible, and reliable the study is, the more unfeasible it is in terms of the volume of observations that you have to make: the more feasible, more subjective the work, and the more open to suspicion of contamination.

A variation on the use of key informants for the location of behavior settings might be to treat the sample 500 respondents as key informants by asking each where their behavior settings are, and to obtain similar information it can be determined which ones have accurate knowledge of the area based on whether discrepancies exist between their settings and the consensus. It also may obtain their view of the extent of their participation in the neighborhood.

The CPSP research objective here, which is to assess the functional interdependence, or interface, or level of integration of the environment, probably would not find identification of respondents as important as observing what goes on in behavior settings. A prime need is to refine the operations presently employed to distinguish areas on this dimension. Presently there are ten criteria, and the hope is to achieve something more precise on the level of a numerical score. Counterfoil methods would be useful and behavior settings might be the way to do it; however, they would be more meaningful if knowledge was obtainable not only of their number but about the kind of behavior in each as well. It isn't necessary to go into the motives, attitudes, and emotions of people here, particularly since it is better to keep the variable concerned with integration-disintegration separate from those variables dependent on how people feel.

There is a need to specify the trains of behavior that are being looked for, and after that ask in what kinds of behavioral settings one should look for those. If the concern is with behavior that is indicative of integration or disintegration, then one looks for places where this is likely to occur. But one must also have a reason for looking. The climate of a big city may encourage anonymity; this may be a parameter in an urban-rural comparison, but it is not a variable unless the research at hand has a hypothesis that it is or is not conducive to mental health. The logic of the study doesn't call for a representative sample of behavior settings, what we need to know is which ones are relevant.

The foregoing summarizes the basic ideas presented in this seminar. Now, three of the presenters, Herbert Gans, Ph.D., Alexander H. Leighton, M.D., and John Gulick, Ph.D., comment on their ideas.

PRESENTER: HERBERT GANS, Ph.D.

Gans: I am skeptical about the concept of community. Even the West End of Boston, which I called an urban village, was in many ways just a collection of families living next to each other. Levittown, a big suburban development near Philadelphia, is very different from the adjacent towns, so that looking at it from the outside, it appears to be a community. Looking at it from the inside, however, the relation of the residents to that mythical entity called Levittown is pretty tenuous. Still, one can use the term community to describe this relation, but one must do it in several senses.

First, there are socio-metric communities on every block. Generally speaking, they cover the four houses on either side of one's own house, and within this small area people relate to some but not all of their neighbors, exchanging visits and mutual aid in the traditional ways associated with "community." Second, there is the political and administrative entity called Levittown, which is governed by elected officials. Many of the decisions of these officials affect only a few residents, but some affect many of the residents. For example, when school taxes rose sharply, the less affluent residents were squeezed financially; they protested and voted elected officials out of office. Such events are rare, however. Third, there is the network of the voluntary associations, which concern a small number of active people and provide some services to the nonmember population. This network has some ties with political organizations, and individual associations compete with each other in various ways, but the area in which they function could be called the community. However, it coincides, for most organizations, with the community governed by the elected officials.

Nevertheless, it is difficult to trace any aspect of community other than these that really has a major impact on people, and even these three probably have a minimal impact on most people. It would be difficult to document that these aspects of community cause stress. In some instances they do; the sociometric community is stressful to the people who are left out of it, who are ignored by their neighbors; the political community can create stresses for people who suffer hardship from its decisions; the associational community may result in stress for the handful of people who do the major share of "community activity."

But Levittown is a bedroom community and does not significantly affect the economic welfare of its residents. Higher taxes or mortgage payments can squeeze family finances, but Levittown does not bring about unemployment, or a raise, or a better job; these changes come from the national economy and from the regional economy of which Levittown is a part.

I suspect that Levittown is not as different from New York as one might think. Of course, New York is an important economic entity; it can affect people's jobs and thus their daily life. Also, it is a rapidly changing community; the processes of invasion and succession bring about neighborhood changes which benefit some and cost others. The political community probably has most impact on the poor and especially those outside the labor force; it determines which areas are to be torn down for urban renewal and, more important, how much will be given in public assistance payments.

Murphy: Well, I understand that you got interested in studying "West End" with relation to the fact that it was going to be a relocated area. I don't think that any of us in trying to think through the problem of how we're going to study this segment of the urban environment are committed to the constant community, but we have spent a lot of time trying to decide whether we should use the place where people live, in other words, the residential area as a place to begin the study.

This must have come up in your mind, too, in terms of—is it efficient to walk around the block and see what the people do on the street, how they lean out of windows?

Gans: No, the West End just happened to be available to study, and before I knew it I was spending time on urban renewal and the impact of relocation. I would agree that in any community, the basic unit is going to be the family, unless you happen to be studying professors, and in that instance, there seems to be some doubt about whether the family or the job is the principal focus in their lives.

For the working class and the lower middle class, the job is most often just a place to make money, to have some more companionship, to get away from the family, to get, possibly, hopefully, some job satisfaction.

In Levittown, the most important units are home and the family, and not the job. In the "West End" it wasn't the home so much because the male-female relationships were much more segregated. Home was not a major physical center for the family.

Langner: What about religion? Talking about all these other institutions, are the people let's say in Levittown organized around their religious groups?

Gans: Some of them. The Jews organized very quickly around their synagogues. Once they organized, however, they stopped attending them. I don't think religion had much to do with the organization of the synagogues; they were ethnic centers. The synagogue has been a traditional ethnic center.

The fundamental Baptists, of whom there are quite a few in Levittown, really live their lives around the church, with services on

Sunday and another prayer meeting on Wednesday night. Also, most of their social contacts are with other church members because they don't drink, they don't smoke, and they disagree on other issues with their neighbors.

The Irish, German, and Italian Catholics go to church almost every Sunday morning. The other Protestants go less often. There is, however, always a small core of people who adopt the church as their organization or their club, and work for it.

For the large majority, the church is not crucial in their lives, though some of the ethnic beliefs are of importance. (I was curious about the impact of secularization that was mentioned in the Stirling papers. I was wondering whether this was a transitional phenomenon that was founded in New York City or other American towns twenty-five, thirty years ago.)

Today most communities are effectively securlarized. Even though most people say they believe in God, this belief doesn't have much relevance to what else they are doing. They have overcome the strains of the culture shift from sacred to secular without too much difficulty.
Freydberg: Let me raise a strange issue in relation to this. In effect, you don't really feel a sense, among these people, of the importance of community in their lives. And yet an incident was reported in the newspapers last week; a group of the thirty-eight people in a part of New York, in Queens, observed someone being murdered and none of them took any action whatever.

Now if something in a community of this sort is going on, perhaps this is a curvilinear relationship as you get to a certain level of integration, and causes an indifference in it. Perhaps this is a phenomenon in certain urban areas, perhaps not. It's something we find very hard to understand.
Fales: I think we can draw another parallel, such as this white man from Idaho who was murdered in Harlem. It certainly drew a lot of people together, at least after his death, in some sort of recognition of his meaning in the community.

I don't think it has anything to do with our study, but there is another point I thought I'd raise: Do we want to just try to pre-associate with those in the community; or should we try to think that our purpose here is to try to draw the sample?

II. PRESENTER: ALEXANDER H. LEIGHTON, M.D.

A. Leighton: Let me interject an observation at this point with regard to the community concept in the Nova Scotia study. I think Dr. Chein said virtually everything that covers that orientation with his emphasis on the interdependence.

I want to restate it a little bit, perhaps for emphasis. First of all there isn't any question as to whether these are communities. We're using the word community to refer to a collection of people who geographically live together, and it doesn't say anthing about their attitudes toward altruism or toward dealing with a feeling of "we-ness." But people who live together in a geographical way with distance separating them from other groups have certain interdependent characteristics. They are interdependent in terms of the economy, for instance, within the community. There is, of course, economic dependence of that community on the larger society and on other communities around which have various relationships to each other economically, but setting that aside, within the geographic boundary of this community (and the Nova Scotia community would be different I suppose, from Levittown), there is a high degree of economic interdependence on the part of the people there.

What happens to A, whether it relates to B or not, is going to have an effect on B. Secondly there is a high interdependence among the people there for protection, protection such as the law, which is many miles away from these communities.

Very often they have volunteer or deputy police who are defined by some kind of community council. But the real, effective law and order is obtained on an informal basis by the kind of behavior that people have toward each other, first of all, verbal sanctions of various sorts, and if things go too far, or before they go too far, actual intervention.

Usually the last thing they do is call in the formal law organization, although this may happen on occasion. But there is mutual protection from interpersonal hostilities or interpersonal behavior. There are limits to what people are free to do to each other, so that an individual feels that in a certain respect he is protected in this situation.

This doesn't necessarily involve any attitudes of altruism or anything of this sort, but it is the reality of the situation. Secondly, there is interdependence toward protection against disease, fire, accidents, and acts of God; fire in this part of the world is fairly important. You can always count on the community turning out in such a case and even helping to build a house afterwards if it is necessary.

The doing of these things, again, does not depend on these people liking each other, or even liking the community. They may say it's a hell of a place to live, but they nevertheless perform these functions when the occasion arises.

Thirdly, I'd stress disease, which goes into this too, as I think I mentioned. The garbage on the steps that Dr. Chein mentioned would be quite an important thing. You can get away with a certain amount of behavior, but not if you go beyond a certain point in acts which threaten the rest of the community with the spread of disease, such as letting refuse get into the drinking water. Anybody that goes throwing dead cats into other people's wells is going to get clobbered by the community sooner or later.

So there is protection against disease as part of this pattern, and then there is the business of education. One of the webs of interdependence in a community is the whole process of inducting children into the educational system.

Now, there is a strong interference from the outside in this, in that the schools are provincial; but nevertheless the local school board is the one that hires and fires the teacher and sets the tone, and what goes on in the local schools is very much influenced by them.

So the emotional and social needs of individuals are met by various local clubs, organizations, etc., all down the line. Through all of this, cutting across it in a different dimension, is the dimension of communication, of interpersonal interactions, from roadways and paths, to telephones—channels whereby people do communicate with each other so that these various functions get performed as the need arises.

This is all without any reference to feeling, necessarily, that they are all devoted to their community. Within the framework of community to community, these items I've just been outlining may be performed badly or they may be performed well, but they are performed purely from a functional point of view.

This gets into what we have in mind when we talk about disintegration of the community, wherein functions of this sort are constantly misfiring, are self-defeating, and don't necessarily come off. Whereas in a well-integrated community they get done, whatever may be the fabric or sentiments on which they rest.

In one of the areas of research is the question of what kinds of sentiments do different kinds of communities have who are performing these functions badly or well. An item of considerable interest with regard to this situation is the suggestion that this may be something that once existed in upstate New York or in other parts of the country and no longer does. I think this is very opposite.

Personally I think it still exists in large areas of upstate New York, as well as in Nova Scotia. But I think you can look at the history of the last fifty years and see very plainly what's happening; because all of these things I've mentioned, such as economics, self-protection, education, and so on, fifty years ago were far more community-contained than they are now. One of the progressive things for instance, was that the local village or town was entirely responsible for its roads.

Nowadays the roads are taken care of by the provincial department of highways, and the main contribution of the community is the tax that they pay, whether they like it or not.

So any decisions about what kinds of roads the community has, have been tenuated in terms of the functions that the community can perform. You can go down the list of things the community council now does and compare them with what the community council did fifty years ago, and you'll see it's a pale ghost of what it used to be because of the professionalization of the services that exist in education, highways, health, and so on.

It's still there, it's still acting, and it's still functioning, but it's nothing of what it used to be in terms of local self-determination because of the intervention now of, for instance, the school board, which still hires the teachers but can only hire people that have certain qualifications. And this limits their choice.

And, of course, there are all kinds of things coming in now in terms of provincial money from other sources and with each of these comes the limitation of the amount of choice that the community has.

III. PRESENTER: JOHN GULICK, Ph.D.

Murphy: We are about to begin our afternoon free-for-all. Is it agreeable to the group to begin talking about participant observation and how we might do it in contrasting areas? Perhaps as a lead into that, Dr. Gulick might be willing to tell us a little bit more about how an anthropologist does a study in a Middle Eastern city.

Gulick: I'll be glad to talk about this for a while. I'll try to be brief because I'm a little fearful that some of the material about Tripoli could only be of limited help here—but you will be a better judge of that than I.

It's a city of between 120,000 and 250,000 people. The reason for this wide range is that there has been no census since 1932; this showed a population much smaller than the city obviously has now. I had three estimates from three different responsible officials! I got some absolute, specific figures on the amount of animals slaughtered each day in Beirut and Tripoli, and in Tripoli it is about one-third that of Beirut, which has a population of 500,000 to 600,000. This is the kind of fundamental data problem I was up against.

Tripoli has a built-up area (not counting the port, which is separate) of about one square mile, which is very small. The Tripolitans live either in old houses with many people on one floor, or in high rise apartment houses. Eight stories is pretty high by Tripoli standards.

The apartments are very modern with store fronts in the bottom floors of most of the buildings, so that commercial and residential functions are mixed together. I've noticed the same thing on Second and Third Avenues in New York City, and I've had people jump on me for saying it was peculiar to the Middle East.

But the planners don't seem to think it's a good idea. They'd like to have the commercial separated from the residential. On the contrary, I think it's excellent. It's more convenient, and the streets are better policed because of the store-owners' vigilance.

I knew something about the city before I went there, that it was primarily Moslem with a Christian minority, that it had an old part with arched-over streets and "medieval" buildings, as well as new parts, and so forth. I knew that Tripoli had a reputation for being narrow-minded and conservative.

How I went about getting established was very simple. I had some contacts, friends of friends, whom I went to see as soon as I got there. The first thing that I had to do was to find a place to live, and the solution was to room and board in a home. My original plan was to go from one family to another and thereby place myself in different parts of the city. But this unfortunately did not work out because what happened was that I became established with my hosts and their friends. Middle Easterners have a tendency to be very possessive once they feel you're their friend, and I couldn't get myself out of this household. If I had been cleverer I might have done so, but I am not certain about this. So my original plan for living in different parts of the city for a month or so each fell through.

I worked out from this family. I got to know their friends and friends of their friends. My initial contacts were with Christians, who were outsiders themselves. I used them because the outsider often sees things in the community as a whole that can be helpful. I did get to know some Moslems, but not on the family level of intimacy.

Now, this is the difference—this is where, perhaps, the inapplicability of Tripoli to New York comes in. These people are very, very strongly family centered. That doesn't necessarily mean that the family members love each other, not at all. But they are family centered.

Their recreational activities, such as visits, are family oriented. The family is outwardly very close, and it is considered to be very private. What goes on inside the family is carefully hidden. The old-fashioned house style, which hides the identity of the occupants, is still present even in modern apartment houses. You have to get into the family very deeply in order to learn what life is like to the individual living it. That's pretty hard to do.

I don't know that you necessarily face that problem so much here, where many activities go on outside of the family, as we all know. This is not to say that the family here is necessarily unorganized or functionless, however.

Later on, I did some questionnaire work with people from Tripoli who were university students. Maybe you would like to ask me some questions now.

Voice: What was the purpose of the study?

Gulick: The purpose of the study originally was to discover whether there were differences in group participation, in the sense of responsibility toward larger units than just the family, etc., between migrants to the city and people who have no village ties. The village tie is very important there.

It didn't turn out in the end to be a matter of sharp contrast between village and city orientation, because I discovered that social class variables intervened, and that one's group activities depended very much on what kind of education one had regardless of whether one had village ties; this was true except among the very poor people who, if they were village migrants, retained a sense of village identity very strongly, being clustered together in the city, and so on.

Murphy: Did a sense of identity with Tripoli come out?

Gulick: I haven't worked this out to my satisfaction. I've got some pat answers, but I don't like them. I think that the Moslems who have no village ties have a sense of identity as Moslems and as being non-Beirut people. Tripoli is to Beirut as Buffalo is to New York.

The Tripolitans are known to have a certain reputation and so they have a sense of defensiveness about the identity of the city. Talk about garbage in the streets and not caring about and defacing buildings, projecting from our advantages, you could say that they have no community ties whatsoever. But I'm fearful about this. I start off thinking this way and then I get concerned about it because I feel my own projection is involved.

Murphy: The house type is such that you have to walk in a courtyard in order to get to the family quarters?

Gulick: Well, it depends. The city has been rebuilt extensively. The old house type is like that. But the new house type in which, I would think, the majority of people live, is a multiple-storied apartment house. Some of them are just two stories with the uprights ready for additional stories later on when they get the money. They like to build when they have money, not on credit. There is very little credit available. All the taxes are lower if the building remains unfinished. So in that case you don't walk into any courtyard, you go into an entrance-way.

In a Moslem household they will usher you into a front parlor from which other members of the family can observe you, but not you them. So they've got their protective devices.

Murphy: Since we are interested in observation let's give some thought to what it is that you are able to see in a city. I think it was Dr. Freydberg who suggested that this could be much more effectively done if the apartments in New York City were arranged so that the windows were on the hallway as well as on the outside, and when you walk down the hallways in apartment houses you could look in and see if they are having dinner and what not. I think it is a marvelous idea.

Gulick: There are other things that were involved here, the coffee houses, for instance. There are certain coffee houses in certain areas where people congregate. You can leave packages there and then pick them up later, for example. They are regionally oriented. One's cronies hang out in them. There is also the promenade pattern. And the movie business is very diffuse. But you can get certain cues about groups and networks from the coffee house thing. I think there are parallels to this in New York. As far as private clubs go, there are very, very few. This is all much more simple than it is in our culture as far as I can see.

Langner: Did you sample these behavior settings in some way, or did you simply move through?

Gulick: Frankly I just moved through. I wasn't as thorough as I could have been if I had had a team.

Freydberg: Did you also work in Beirut?

Gulick: No. I had my family there and I commuted. A professor deliberately living in Tripoli would not only be a curiosity, but strange and suspect, because of the attitude: "Who in the world of this sort would live in downtrodden Tripoli?" It was inconvenient in many ways, and, of course, we missed many things. It was a natural way to do it, though, from their point of view. I mean they knew what I was. I always proceed on the basis of what my true identity is.

Freydberg: And they believed you?

Gulick: Oh yes.

Murphy: Do they have telephones?

Gulick: They have telephones, and the telephone book lists approximately 4,000 phones. The phone population is smaller than it is here, and the phone book shows both residences and occupations. Through the phone book I could learn where the people worked, where the business phones were concentrated, and so on. This was a nice windfall that I didn't really expect.

Murphy: It seems to me that we ought to give some thought to telephone messages as involving somewhat the definition of a line for any one person, not only in his home but as he travels throughout the city.

Gulick: This has been done, as a matter of fact. We have a student in North Carolina who took a course that I give on kinship and on social organization, a course in which we talked about these concepts of disintegrating groups, and so on. The matter of communication came up and remained with us, and we reached the conclusion that a great many of the hunches we have about kin behavior assume face-to-face behavior as the only significant kind.

But, as this person pointed out, these days in America the kin groups often use the telephone, telegraph, mail, and that sort of thing as a means of keeping themselves at least in communication and maybe highly integrated. So he went on to investigate this aspect of kinship behavior.

I don't know how you could integrate this type of inquiry into yours, but it is a dimension that I don't think should be forgotten; you might have a nuclear family that appears to have no relatives living nearby, and then you discover they call up Mother fives times a week.

Kinship behavior is an un-mined area, as far as I know.

Gump: There's a woman, I've forgotten her name, who works with Margaret Mead for the Museum of Natural History on a special allocation study, who reported, too, that in certain social agencies in New York they couldn't understand why the dependency need was so apparently kept between mothers and daughters until they applied themselves to the question closely, and saw that very often there were three or four phone calls to Mama a day. Certainly the phone has played an important role in retaining this relationship.

Murphy: Well, these things are adaptable to survey.

Michael: According to their facts it would depend also on who initiates this. I just talked to someone who says he calls his mother every day. And while he says they really don't have very much in common he still calls every day. There are some mothers who insist on this, and sons and daughters who say that if they didn't call Mother every day she would be upset.

Freydberg: As you talk about this area of the phone, I hope there is an Alexander Graham Bell Foundation that can help us with this. It occurs to me that something said earlier by Chein highlights the following: We keep thinking in terms of a man, where he travels to work and travels back home. I have a feeling that this is a vice, that in the city itself, even in the Park Avenue segments, there is a way women get together in Central Park in the safe areas, or in the Bronx around the little parks, or other areas where they wheel their carriages and so forth, that is in itself a nursery on the street—and this is a very active and strong thing in the city, separate from the men.

It may be that the men are just a kind of creature that provide a certain source of fuel, but that the matriarchy which exists in terms of community may be the very strong factor in many streets and neighborhoods of this kind. I know this is true in some areas.

Murphy: Well, the women are inside the houses and the men are on the streets.

Gulick: This is one thing that I would suggest. I don't know how far the participant observation will go; you probably don't know either at this point. But the only thing that I would urge at this juncture, is that at the very least, when you've spotted the individuals you'll be interviewing, pay some attention to the actual locale where the sample is drawn, or the locales from which the individuals are drawn, and have somebody, periodically even, work it out on a seasonal basis and a diurnal basis. This is just to see what goes on in these various streets where your people come from, if you don't want to be in the position of tailing your informants and that sort of thing.

But, although you might get to that (not necessarily tailing but at the very least this accompanying business) do it so that there is some physical niche to be dubbed into the interview, the kind of place it is that they are from, and so on.

I was involved in some research in Greensboro, North Carolina, where this was not done; we didn't have time to do it. All we did was go in and get survey data from people who were bodyless. Nobody ever went and checked on the blocks. The blocks were selected on a random basis, and they did a total saturation of interviews on each block.

The results of this study lacked a good deal, I think, because what I am now urging was not done. Now, this is not saying you ought to stop there. But I think at least it ought to be done, so that you'll know whether a person lives in a high-rise apartment house, or lives in a brownstone and, if so, is he on the front or the back and how many flights does he walk up? Is he near the front corridor where he can see people coming in and out all the time? Is it the kind of a place where the neighbors hang around—this sort of thing. I think this is very important.

Gans: This has to take place before you do anything, before you start your schedule, so you understand the environment that he'll be talking about and so on.

Gulick: Yes, yes.

Freydberg: You have a dimension here that's interesting. The amount of information you have from them about other people will give you some sense of the amount of interaction that goes on in the neighborhood. How much does he know, how many snoops are there?

Murphy: Is that really how to get participant observation or will they know that you'll be doing that sort of thing? Is a lot of that possible to gather in a survey, after which you put your participant observants into a living relationship with them? That is, with whatever leads come out of the idea?

Gans: Well, it's really both. You have a participant observer who goes around and tries to find out all the buildings that are five-story tenements, and then you don't have to ask in the questionnaire how high does it go. If you see the thing you'll ask questions about it, and if you don't see it you might not ask questions about it.

You know if the mothers hang around the grocery store and if at 4 o'clock all the women come out to find out what the winning number was that day. These are things that, if you've initially found out about, you'll think of when you make your schedule. A very simple, short reconnaissance through the neighborhood will give you all kinds of things.

Gulick: Also in the neighborhood where you are interviewing, do there appear to be or do there not appear to be these focal points that might be called "community" nodes? It might be the local tavern or what have you, or it might not.

Murphy: It seems to be that if you're contemplating drawing on whatever can be adapted from the community study approach and being in contact with some city planners, other types of studies that might have some relevance to our problem are the social action programs in the city.

They've had to deal with the problem of whether there is enough community feeling to get something going. I heard a review of urban social action, based on a block in East Harlem, that was done by the American Friends Service Committee. One of the things they did was to put a man and a wife who were both trained social workers into one block (maybe you are all familiar with this study). They began by doing just straight, descriptive ethnography—how many people live in that block? It turned out that there were 3,000 people in one block, which is an awful number. It lets you see what you're going to have to try to deal with. This phenomena that we talked about, of women being the street roamers because they are pushing babies around and what not, was apparently well-exemplified in this block in East Harlem. The wife who was herself a social worker, one day, while there were several other women around her, got them interested in sweeping up the street. And they did sweep it up. Afterwards they got together and had a street party.

The next day, with nobody prompting, everybody shoveled out their apartment doorway, and dust was flying off of rooftops and what not. Apparently there was gradually some sense of wanting to identify with a clean neighborhood.

That's a pretty good indication that in that setting this sense of community developed voluntarily.

Langner: We were doing a study in New York and tried to do a short community study in advance of making out the questionnaire. I must say the material that we got somehow never really got integrated into the questionnaire, I can't say why. But there were several things that came out. For instance, people shopped in stores where other people would go five, six, and seven times a day simply for human contact.

Now the question is do you want to put this kind of thing in the questionnaire? Is it pathology? Or is it simply a very healthy searching out of human contact. Italian families spend a tremendous amount of time in funeral parlors. They spend money on preparing funerals; there is a great deal of involvement with the funeral. A good deal of careful planning by the family organization goes into each death. I'm not talking about the shortage of findings, I'm just talking about an experience now for what it's worth. But these things somehow, I think because of the fact that they were sort of scattered, didn't get integrated with the questionnaire. We couldn't make up questions about it. But somehow there is a finding here and a finding there.

I think if you do a community study you should probably try to focus on specific types of activities that might have some meaning for mental health. I don't know just how you'd go about it.

Gans: This is a very good example, because, you know, we could ask middle-class people, who may have had lots of interaction, five and six times a day with the storekeeper, who their three or four closest friends are, and from their answers realize that some of them never think of the storekeeper as a close friend.

They might, but they might not. But, you'd miss all the interaction by not asking the question. A personal observation here would give you this kind of information.

12

CONCLUDING REMARKS

BERTON H. KAPLAN, Ph. D.

Scientific research is an entry into the endless, not a blind alley; solving one problem, a greater one enters our sight. One answer breeds a multitude of new questions; explanations are merely indications of greater puzzles. Everything hints at something that transcends it; the detail indicates the whole, its idea, its mysterious root. What appears to be a center is but a point on the periphery of another center. The totality of the thing is actual infinity [1].

The purpose of this seminar report has been to highlight the conceptual problem and opportunities of Leighton's theory of integration-disintegration and the application of Leighton's scheme to urban settings. As in Professor Heschel's observations above, the seminar has been devoted to recording the natural history of the development of ideas as exchanged and sharpened in a continuing seminar on a single theme. How do you ask better questions about social process and mental health? How do we develop better calipers to measure these processes?

There are some very important summary questions with which to conclude:

(1) In the spirit of Leighton's framework, how can we best use a theoretical paradigm to hasten and refine the work on social process and mental disorder?

[1] Heschel, A. J. *Between God and Man.* Fritz A. Rothchild (Ed.) New York: Free Press, 1959, P. 46.

(2) What are the criteria for a health social system? What are the criteria of a competent social system?

(3) What are the key social variables that place people at high risk for mental illness?

(4) What are the key social variables that are "protective" against mental illness.

(5) In the spirit of John R. P. French's critique of the integration-disintegration hypothesis (in Chapter 6), what are the critical conditional variables?

(6) What are the best strategies for selecting social units for studying social process and mental illness?

(7) What are the best conceptual strategies for postulating socio- and psychodynamic relationships (e.g., reality conflicts versus dependency need interferences and differences in psychological reactions)?

By making my concluding remarks on the seminar report in this fashion, I am being faithful to an observation by Albert Einstein and Leopold Enfeld:

> The formulation of a problem is often more essential than its solution, which may be merely a matter of mathematical or experimental skill. To raise new questions, new possibilities, to regard old problems through a new angle, requires creative imagination and makes a real advance in science [2].

This entire seminar has been devoted to the spirit of Einstein and Enfeld's observation of seeking to ask more creative and imaginative questions so as to advance our understanding of social process and mental illness.

Taking my cues from S. Y. Agnon, 1966 Nobel Laureate in Literature, I would like to conclude, at the risk of overdoing quotations, from Rabbi Hayyim of Zans, who told the following parables:

[2] Einstein, A. & Enfeld, L. *The Evolution of Physics.* New York: Simon and Schuster, 1942.

A man had been wandering about in a forest for several days, not knowing which was the right way out. Suddenly he saw a man approaching him. His heart was filled with joy. "Now I shall certainly find out which is the right way," he thought to himself. When they neared one another, he asked the man, "Brother, tell me which is the right way. I have been wandering about in this forest for several days." Said the other to him, "Brother, I do not know the way out either. For I, too, have been wandering about here for many, many days. But this I can tell you: do not take the way I have been taking, for that will lead you astray. And now let us look for a new way out together."

Our master added: "So it is with us. One thing I can tell you: the way we have been following this far we ought follow no further, for that way leads one astray. But now let us look for a new way."

There was still another parable that our master used to relate: There was once a poor countrywoman who had many children. They were always begging for food, but she had none to give them. One day she found an egg.

She called her children and said, "Children, children, we've nothing to worry about any more, I've found an egg. And, being a provident woman, I'll not eat the egg, but shall ask my neighbor for permission to set it under her setting hen, until a chick is hatched. For I am a provident woman! And we'll not eat the chick, but will set her on eggs, and the eggs will hatch into chickens. And the chickens in their turn will hatch many eggs, and we'll have many chickens and many eggs. But I'm a provident woman, I am! I'll not eat the chickens and not eat the eggs, but shall sell them and buy me a heifer. And I'll not eat the heifer, but shall raise it to a cow, and not eat the cow until it calves. And I'll not eat it then, either, and we'll have cows and calves. For I'm a provident woman! And I'll sell the cows and the calves and buy a field, and we'll have fields and cows and we won't need anything any more!"

The countrywoman was speaking in this fashion and playing with the egg, when it fell out of her hands and broke. Said our master: "That is how we are. When the holy days arrive, every person resolves to do Teshuvah, thinking in his heart, 'I'll do this, and I'll do that.' But the

days slip by in mere deliberation, and thought doesn't lead
to action, and what is worse, the person who made the
resolution may fall even lower . . . . [3]

This seminar report has been written in the spirt of the first parable,
the wish to either stay out of the woods or to make sure we do not go
astray in our pursuit of effective scientific formulations. And as in the
second parable of the woman with the egg, I feel that the publication of
the seminar results will speed us along and make our work more
productive.

[3] Agnon, S. Y. *Days of Awe.* New York: Schocken Books, Inc., 1948, P. 22.